Journey to Inception of Life
A Guide to
ART Laboratory Techniques

Journey to Inception of Life
A Guide to
ART Laboratory Techniques

Chandan Vijay Salunke
PhD
Managing Director
Kasturi ReproAssist Concepts LLP
Panjim, Goa, India

Shravani Kanakdas Parker
MSc
Executive Director
Kasturi ReproAssist Concepts LLP
Panjim, Goa, India

Foreword
Kedarnath Manohar Padte

JAYPEE

JAYPEE BROTHERS MEDICAL PUBLISHERS
The Health Sciences Publisher
New Delhi | London

Jaypee Brothers Medical Publishers (P) Ltd

Headquarters

Jaypee Brothers Medical Publishers (P) Ltd
EMCA House, 23/23-B
Ansari Road, Daryaganj
New Delhi 110 002, India
Landline: +91-11-23272143, +91-11-23272703
+91-11-23282021, +91-11-23245672
Email: jaypee@jaypeebrothers.com

Corporate Office

Jaypee Brothers Medical Publishers (P) Ltd
4838/24, Ansari Road, Daryaganj
New Delhi 110 002, India
Phone: +91-11-43574357
Fax: +91-11-43574314
Email: jaypee@jaypeebrothers.com

Overseas Office

JP Medical Ltd.
83, Victoria Street, London
SW1H 0HW (UK)
Phone: +44 20 3170 8910
Fax: +44 (0)20 3008 6180
Email: info@jpmedpub.com

Website: www.jaypeebrothers.com
Website: www.jaypeedigital.com

Inquiries for bulk sales may be solicited at: jaypee@jaypeebrothers.com

Journey to Inception of Life: A Guide to ART Laboratory Techniques

First Edition: **2025**

ISBN: 978-93-6616-905-7

Printed at: Samrat Offset Pvt. Ltd.

Dedication

In loving memory of Jayant Kamat.

A visionary in IVF, Dr Kamat's compassion, dedication and unwavering pursuit of excellence brought hope to countless families and shaped the future of reproductive medicine. His life's work continues to inspire and his legacy lives on in every life he touched and every miracle he made possible.

Foreword

Two streams merged to form a river, clear crystal, pure, and bubbly. Eventually, gathering force turned into a river of knowledge that caused a delta in assisted reproductive technology (ART), before merging into the "Ocean" of knowledge of assisted reproduction. Dr Chandan Vijay Salunke and Shravani Kanakdas Parker have done exactly that and are continuing to course their path from ripples into waves.

As I reflect on the remarkable advancements in the field of ART, I am filled with a deep sense of pride and admiration for the two brilliant minds behind this book. Having known both of the authors for many years, I consider them not only esteemed colleagues but also like my own children, each bringing a unique perspective and wealth of experience to the work you now hold in your hands.

Their work has always been rooted in the principles of precision, care, and a deep respect for the human life they help create. Through this book, they generously share their wealth of experience, providing invaluable insights that will undoubtedly guide practitioners across the globe. Their dedication to continuous learning and the application of the latest technologies in ART reflects the spirit of progress that is vital to the advancement of our field. I have watched them grow into confident, knowledgeable professionals, and it brings me great satisfaction to see their contributions taking shape within these pages.

To me, this book is not just a scientific resource; it is a reflection of a journey—a journey of knowledge, growth, and the relentless pursuit of helping others realize the dream of parenthood. The authors have taken complex topics and broken them down into clear, accessible content that will benefit not only seasoned professionals but also those entering the field of ART for the first time.

As someone who has had the privilege of guiding and working with both of these remarkable individuals, I can say with certainty that their collaboration represents the perfect balance between experience and innovation. Their shared values of dedication, compassion, and excellence resonate through every chapter of this book.

I am honored to present this work to you, confident that it will serve as an indispensable guide in the ever-evolving field of reproductive medicine. May it inspire, inform, and, most importantly, enhance the lives of countless families worldwide.

Kedarnath Manohar Padte
MBBS DGO MD (Obs-Gyn) DNB FICS
Dip in Endoscopic Surgery Dip in IVF and ICSI
Director
Dr Kedar's Maternity, Infertility
and Surgical Hospital
Panjim, Goa, India

Preface

The creation of this book has been a journey that reflects our passion, dedication, and shared experiences in the ever-evolving field of embryology. This work stands as both a personal and a professional milestone for us, representing the culmination of years spent to understand and improve the intricate processes that form the foundation of assisted reproductive technology (ART).

Writing this book has been born out of a desire to contribute meaningfully to the ART community. We recognize that the science of reproductive medicine is as much about human hope and aspiration as it is about technical precision. Our aim has been to provide a resource that speaks not only to the mechanics of embryology but also to the profound impact that this work has on the lives of those seeking to create a new life.

This book is more than a collection of facts and protocols; it is a reflection of the lessons we have learned over years of practice and observation. We are indebted to our mentors, colleagues, and students—each of whom has contributed to the knowledge and understanding we now share. It is with deep gratitude and respect that we offer this work to the broader community, in the hope that it will inspire and guide future practitioners on their own journeys.

We invite you to explore these pages with the same curiosity and commitment that we have brought to our work, and we trust that this book will serve as a valuable companion in your pursuit of excellence in embryology.

Chandan Vijay Salunke
Shravani Kanakdas Parker

Acknowledgments

As we bring this book to completion, we are filled with immense gratitude for the many people who have supported and guided us throughout this journey. The process of writing this book has been both challenging and rewarding, and we could not have accomplished it without the encouragement, wisdom, and love of those around us.

We are also deeply indebted to our mentors and colleagues in the field of embryology. Your expertise, insight, and generosity in sharing knowledge have been invaluable in shaping our understanding of this complex field.

To our parents, friends, and families, your patience and unwavering support have been invaluable throughout this journey. Thank you for your understanding and for standing by us at every stage. Your love has provided us with comfort and motivation, and for that, we are deeply grateful.

Finally, we extend our gratitude to the many patients and families who have trusted us with their hopes and dreams. It is your stories, resilience, and courage that inspire us to push the boundaries of science and continue striving for excellence in the field of reproductive medicine.

This book is a reflection of all the people who have touched our lives and shaped our journey, and for that, we are forever grateful.

Contents

1 CHAPTER

Introduction to Assisted Reproductive Technology Laboratory

INTRODUCTION

The Assisted reproductive technology (ART) laboratory represents a cornerstone of modern fertility treatments, facilitating advanced techniques such as in vitro fertilization (IVF), intracytoplasmic sperm injection (ICSI), and preimplantation genetic testing. By combining cutting-edge infrastructure with precise methodologies, ART laboratories address various infertility challenges, enable genetic screening, and support fertility preservation.

The evolution of ART has transformed reproductive medicine globally, with significant contributions from pioneers and technological advancements. India's journey in ART underscores its growing prominence in providing innovative fertility solutions and expanding access to reproductive healthcare.

EVOLUTION OF ASSISTED REPRODUCTIVE TECHNOLOGY

Historical Milestones in Assisted Reproductive Technology

Assisted reproductive technology (ART) has made remarkable progress since its inception. The journey began with the birth of Louise Brown, the first successful in vitro fertilization (IVF) baby, in 1978, marking a revolutionary advancement in reproductive medicine.[1] This breakthrough paved the way for numerous innovations and techniques in ART.

In the 1980s and 1990s, techniques such as gamete intrafallopian transfer (GIFT) and zygote intrafallopian transfer (ZIFT) were developed. GIFT, introduced in 1984, involves placing sperm and eggs into the fallopian tubes for natural fertilization.[2] ZIFT, introduced shortly after, involves transferring fertilized zygotes into the fallopian tubes.[3]

Another significant milestone was the introduction of intracytoplasmic sperm injection (ICSI) in 1992, which involves the direct injection of a single sperm into an egg, offering a key solution for male infertility.[4] This technique has become a standard procedure in ART since then **(Table 1)**.

The 21st century has witnessed advancements in preimplantation genetic diagnosis (PGD) and preimplantation genetic screening (PGS), allowing for genetic testing of embryos before implantation, thereby identifying genetic disorders and improving IVF success rates.[5]

INDIAN SCENARIO

The Indian landscape of ART has witnessed a transformative journey over the past few decades. With the increasing prevalence of infertility, ART has emerged as a critical solution for many couples across the country. The first successful IVF procedure in India

TABLE 1: Key milestones in assisted reproductive technology (ART) development.

Year	*Milestone*	*Description*
1978	First IVF baby	Louise Brown, the world's first baby conceived via in vitro fertilization (IVF), was born in the UK
1984	Introduction of gamete intrafallopian transfer (GIFT)	GIFT involves transferring eggs and sperm directly into a woman's fallopian tubes
1986	Introduction of zygote intrafallopian transfer (ZIFT)	ZIFT involves fertilizing the egg outside the body and then placing the resulting zygote into the fallopian tube
1992	Introduction of intracytoplasmic sperm injection (ICSI)	ICSI involves injecting a single sperm directly into an egg, significantly improving fertilization rates for male infertility
1990	First successful preimplantation genetic diagnosis (PGD)	PGD is used to screen embryos for genetic diseases before implantation and pregnancy
1999	Introduction of preimplantation genetic screening (PGS)	PGS is used to screen embryos for chromosomal normality, increasing the success rates of IVF by selecting embryos with the correct number of chromosomes

was a monumental milestone, marking the beginning of a new era in reproductive medicine. The country's fertility industry has since grown exponentially, with numerous clinics offering advanced ART services, making India one of the leading destinations for fertility treatments globally.

First In Vitro Fertilization Baby

India's first IVF baby, Kanupriya Agarwal, fondly known as Durga, was born on October 3, 1978, just months after the birth of Louise Brown, the world's first IVF baby. This historic event was the result of the pioneering work of Dr Subhash Mukhopadhyay, a brilliant but often overlooked scientist in the global narrative of IVF history. Despite the lack of recognition during his lifetime, Dr Mukhopadhyay's contribution to the field of reproductive medicine remains a cornerstone of India's ART journey.

Her birth also laid the foundation for further research and development in the field of ART in India, leading to the establishment of numerous fertility clinics and research centers across the country. Durga's birth symbolizes the triumph of science and perseverance and continues to inspire advancements in reproductive health in India.

PETRI DISH: CRADLE OF LIFE

- The Petri dish is an essential tool in IVF procedures, named after the German bacteriologist Julius Richard Petri, who invented it in 1887. It is a shallow, circular dish made from glass or plastic, commonly used to culture cells, including embryos during IVF.
- In the context of IVF, the Petri dish provides a controlled environment where the oocytes (eggs) and sperm can interact. This setup mimics natural fertilization conditions but allows for direct observation and intervention if necessary.
- The dish is specifically designed to maintain optimal conditions for fertilization, including the appropriate pH, temperature, and gas composition. The culture medium within the dish supports the viability and development of the embryo before it is transferred to the uterus.

OVERVIEW OF COMMON ASSISTED REPRODUCTIVE TECHNOLOGY PROCEDURES

The ART encompasses various procedures addressing different infertility causes. Key procedures include:

- *IVF:* It involves retrieving eggs from the ovaries, fertilizing them with sperm in a lab, and transferring the resulting embryos into the uterus. IVF addresses issues like tubal factor infertility, endometriosis, and unexplained infertility.[6]
- *ICSI:* It is a specialized form of IVF focusing on male infertility, involving the injection of a single sperm into an egg, followed by embryo transfer.[4]
- *GIFT:* In this, eggs and sperm are placed into the fallopian tubes, allowing natural fertilization within the body.[2]
- *ZIFT:* It is similar to GIFT but fertilization occurs in the lab, and the resulting zygote is placed into the fallopian tubes.[3]
- *PGD and PGS:* It is genetic testing of embryos before implantation to identify genetic abnormalities. It is used to prevent genetic disorders and improve implantation rates.[5]
- *Cryopreservation:* It is the process of freezing eggs, sperm, or embryos for future use, particularly useful for patients undergoing medical treatments that may affect reproductive capabilities.[6]

IMPORTANCE OF ASSISTED REPRODUCTIVE TECHNOLOGY IN MODERN MEDICINE

Role in Treating Infertility

Infertility affects about 10–15% of couples globally.[7] ART provides crucial solutions for these couples, offering a range of procedures tailored to specific infertility issues. IVF bypasses tubal blockages, while ICSI addresses severe male infertility by enabling fertilization despite low sperm count or poor sperm quality.[4] ART techniques like PGD and PGS allow couples with genetic disorders to have healthy offspring, reducing the risk of inherited conditions.[5]

Success Rates and Societal Impact

Assisted reproductive technology success rates have significantly improved due to technological advancements. The live birth rate for IVF cycles using fresh embryos in women under 35 is about 45% per cycle.[8] This rate decreases with advancing maternal age but shows an upward trend with continuous ART improvements.

Assisted reproductive technology has also impacted societal demographics, particularly in countries with declining birth rates, enabling couples to have children later in life and counteracting trends in delayed childbearing.[9] Today, fertility preservation options like egg freezing offer women greater flexibility in balancing personal and professional lives.[10]

CONCLUSION

Assisted reproductive technology laboratories are at the heart of modern fertility treatments, offering advanced solutions like IVF, ICSI, and genetic testing to help individuals and couples overcome infertility. These laboratories combine cutting-edge technology, precise protocols, and expert care to achieve the best possible outcomes. Their evolution has not only transformed reproductive medicine globally but also had a profound impact in India, where significant advancements have expanded access to innovative fertility treatments. By continually driving research and embracing new techniques, ART laboratories remain a beacon of hope for those seeking to build families, shaping thc futurc of rcproductivc healthcare.

REFERENCES

1. Edwards RG. The bumpy road to human in vitro fertilization. Nat Med. 2001;7(10):1091-4.
2. Asch RH, Ellsworth LR, Balmaceda JP, Wong PC. Pregnancy after translaparoscopic gamete intrafallopian transfer. Lancet. 1984;2(8410):1034-5.
3. Devroey P, Van Steirteghem AC, Nagy Z, Camus M. Zygote intrafallopian transfer (ZIFT): A new approach to tubal infertility. BJOG. 1896;93(9):873-6.
4. Palermo G, Joris H, Devroey P, Van Steirteghem AC. Pregnancies after intracytoplasmic injection of single spermatozoon into an oocyte. Lancet. 1992;340(8810):17-8.
5. Harper JC, Coonen E, Handyside AH, Paulsen H, De Rycke M, Sermon K, Thornhill AR. The evolution of PGD and PGS. Human Reproduction Update. 2010;16(1):115-23.
6. Practice Committee of the American Society for Reproductive Medicine. Evaluation and treatment of endometriosis: A committee opinion. Fertil Steril. 2012;98(4):713-22.
7. Mascarenhas MN, Flaxman SR, Boerma T, Vanderpoel S, Stevens GA. National, regional, and global trends in infertility prevalence since 1990: A systematic analysis of 277 health surveys. PLOS Med. 2012;9(12):e1001356.
8. Society for Assisted Reproductive Technology (SART). (2020). National Summary Report for 2018. [online]. Available from https://www.sartcorsonline.com/rptCSR_PublicMultYear.aspx?ClinicPKID=0 [Last accessed November, 2024].
9. Schmidt L, Sobotka T, Bentzen JG, Nyboe Andersen A. Demographic and medical consequences of the postponement of parenthood. Hum Reprod Update. 2012; 18(1):29-43.
10. Practice Committee of the American Society for Reproductive Medicine. Fertility preservation in patients undergoing gonadotoxic therapy or gonadectomy: A committee opinion. Fertil Steril. 2013; 100(5): 1214-23.

CHAPTER 2

Setting Up an Assisted Reproductive Technology Laboratory

INTRODUCTION

Setting up an Assisted Reproductive Technology (ART) laboratory is a complex yet essential process that lays the foundation for successful reproductive treatments. Every detail matters, from designing a layout that ensures efficiency and sterility to creating an environment that supports the delicate handling of gametes and embryos. The laboratory must be carefully organized into specific zones to minimize contamination and enhance workflow, while factors like temperature, humidity, and air quality need to be consistently monitored and controlled. This guide explores the critical elements of building a functional and safe ART laboratory, including the selection of advanced equipment, maintaining cleanliness, and adhering to safety standards, to provide the best possible outcomes for patients.

LABORATORY DESIGN AND LAYOUT

Key Considerations for Laboratory Design

The design of an assisted reproductive technology (ART) laboratory is crucial for functionality, efficiency, and compliance with regulatory standards. In vitro fertilization (IVF) setup is recommended away from vibrations, i.e., away from main roads, lifts, loud generators, etc. A specific pattern of design is worked out, so as to avoid direct lights, air, and temperature exposures to ultra-sterile areas. The sections are divided into unsterile, partial sterile, semi-sterile, and ultra-sterile zones. Recommended flow of the rooms is semen collection room, buffer zone, wash area, changing room, andrology laboratory, insemination room, second buffer, second wash, second changing room, cryopreservation room, buffer, and IVF operation theater (OT) followed by IVF laboratory **(Fig. 1)**.

Key considerations include:

- *Workflow optimization:*
    - *Strategic placement:* Workstations and equipment should be strategically placed to minimize unnecessary steps and enhance productivity. For example, placing embryo workstations near incubators reduces handling time and potential contamination.[1] Movement of gametes and embryos in less than one-meter area gives excellent outcomes.
    - *Zoning:* Separate areas for different processes (e.g., gamete handling and embryo culture) to prevent cross-contamination and ensure smooth workflow. Cryo-room should exactly be adjacent to IVF lab as well as close to main entrance for comfortable refilling of liquid nitrogen near buffer area.
- *Environmental control:*
    - *Temperature and humidity:* Constant temperature (37°C) and humidity (45–55%) control are crucial for optimal conditions. Humidity remains crucial

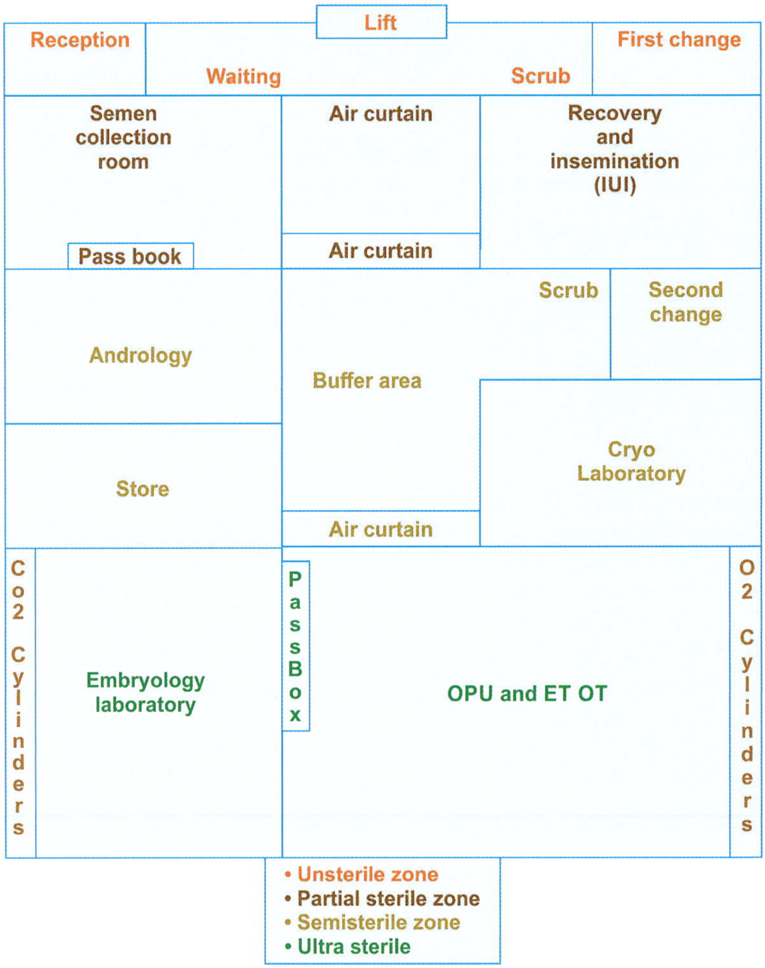

Fig. 1: Optimal lab design: Diagrammatic representation of ideal "S" and "C" Layouts. (ET: embryo transfer; IUI: intrauterine insemination; OT: operation theater OPU: ovum pickup)

factor that protects the optical lenses of the microscopes. Use sensors and automated systems for consistent environmental parameters.[2]

- *Air quality:* High-efficiency particulate air (HEPA) filters and positive pressure systems maintain air purity. Regular air quality testing should be performed to monitor particulate levels and ensure compliance with standards. Air purifiers are also handy in maintaining the ultra-sterile conditions.
- *Light exposure:* Use low-intensity, nonfluorescent lighting to prevent damage to gametes and embryos. Usually warm-white light is additionally used on floors to avoid direct exposure of sample dishes.

▪ *Sterility and Cleanliness:*
  - *Materials and finishes:* Use nonporous surfaces such as stainless steel or Corian for worktops and seamless flooring for easy cleaning and sterilization.[3] Joint-free surfaces are of

ultimate importance that avoid blind spots and hidden area.

- *Waste disposal systems:* Implement proper systems for biological and chemical waste disposal. Use autoclavable waste containers and ensure regular waste removal. Color coding of waste bins can be useful to maintain better disposal.

- *Safety:*
    - *Ergonomic workstations:* Design workstations to prevent repetitive strain injuries, including adjustable chairs and microscopes.[4] 0.3 μm filters, integrated heating, and vibration-noise-free models are of high importance. Integrated recording system with wire-free camera could be an addition.
    - *Ventilation systems:* Adequate ventilation removes harmful fumes, particularly in areas where volatile chemicals are used. External air handling systems, portable air filters, air showers, and air purifiers are also used to maintain sterility in the air. Dehumidification systems and heating coils along with air handling unit (AHU) may be helpful.
    - *Hazardous material storage:* Secure storage areas for hazardous materials with clear labeling and restricted access should be used.

Essential Zones: Reception, Collection, Laboratory, and Recovery Areas

Essential zones include the following:

- *Reception area:*
    - *Privacy:* Ensure privacy for patient registration and consultation with soundproof rooms and discrete entrances/exits.[5]
    - *Comfort:* Provide comfortable seating, calming decor, and informative literature to enhance the patient experience.
- *Collection area:*
    - *Facilities:* Equip soundproof private rooms for semen collection with appropriate furniture and distractions from stress (e.g., magazines and TV).
    - *Immediate processing:* Implement procedures for immediate labeling and processing to maintain sample integrity.[3]
- *Laboratory area:*
    - *Subdivisions:* There should be sections for semen analysis, oocyte retrieval, fertilization, and embryo culture each adhering to strict environmental and sterility standards.[1]
    - *Cleanroom standards should be* International Organization for Standardization (ISO) Class 7 or higher for embryo handling areas to minimize contamination.
- *Recovery area:*
    - *Comfort and monitoring:* Provide comfortable beds, privacy curtains, and vital sign monitoring equipment to ensure patient safety postprocedure.[5]

EQUIPMENT AND INSTRUMENTATION

Basic and Advanced Laboratory Equipment

- *Basic equipment:*
    - *Microscopes:* Inverted microscopes for IVF and intracytoplasmic sperm injection (ICSI) procedures with high-magnification and high-resolution models for detailed analysis are needed.[6] The andrology laboratory should be equipped with a compound

microscope, with an additional recording system that may be beneficial for showing live samples to patients. The embryology laboratory requires at least two microscopes: An inverted microscope for micromanipulation and a stereo-zoom microscope for the workstation. Wireless cameras and recording systems are invaluable for research, training, and recordkeeping purposes.

- *Incubators for* precise control of temperature, humidity, and gas concentrations, with integrated alarms for deviations in environmental parameters are required.[7] Minimum three CO_2 incubators are required, one for andrology and two for embryology laboratory. In an embryology lab, it is optimal to designate one incubator as a working incubator for media and dishes, while dedicating another specifically for embryo culture to minimize disturbances. Additional incubators can be allocated for dedicated Day 3 and Day 5 cultures. The inclusion of tri-gas incubators may further enhance culture conditions.
- *Centrifuges are required for* sperm preparation techniques like density gradient centrifugation and swim-up methods with programmable speed settings and safety features.[8] Temperature-controlled centrifuges are also utilized. The selection of a centrifuge is typically based on its capacity, ease of use, and the presence of a vibration-free, silent motor.
- *Laminar flow hoods:* Provide Class II biosafety cabinet conditions for handling gametes and embryos, protecting them from contamination.[2] Filters with a 0.3 μm diameter, integrated heating, and vibration-free, noise-free models are essential features to consider. An integrated recording system with a wireless camera can be a valuable addition. Opting for stainless steel surfaces over powder-coated ones is advantageous for long-term durability.

- *Advanced equipment:*
  - *Time-lapse imaging systems:* Enable continuous monitoring of embryo development without disturbing culture conditions. Use algorithms for automated embryo assessment to improve selection accuracy.[9] This system minimizes embryo exposure and includes automation for selecting embryos for transfer. It allows differentiation of the developmental potential among groups of embryos, making it a valuable tool for research purposes.
  - *Laser systems should be used* for assisted hatching and embryo biopsy, enhancing precision, and reducing potential damage to embryos with low-power lasers for minimal invasiveness.[10] Measuring the thickness of the zona pellucida can be a useful tool for selecting embryos and assisting hatching, particularly for embryos with a thicker zona.
  - *Cryopreservation equipment:* Programmable freezers and storage tanks for vitrification and long-term storage of gametes and embryos are helpful. Ensure that cryoprotectants are used to prevent ice formation.[11]

Importance of Maintaining and Calibrating Equipment

- *Routine cleaning:* Ensure daily cleaning protocols for surfaces, incubators, and laminar flow hoods using appropriate disinfectants[2]

- *Scheduled maintenance:* Regular servicing of equipment by qualified technicians should be done to identify and fix issues preemptively. Maintenance contracts with manufacturers ensure timely service.[7]
- *Calibration:* Regular calibration of instruments like pipettes, microscopes, and incubators to ensure precision using certified calibration standards and documentation of calibration records are essential.[6]

EQUIPMENT MAINTENANCE AND LABORATORY CLEANLINESS

Lab Environment and Equipment Maintenance

The lab environment and equipment maintenance include:

- *Daily and monthly cleaning:* Rigorous cleaning of surfaces, equipment, and floors with volatile organic compounds (VOC)-free disinfectants.
- *Equipment logs:* Maintain logs for all equipment detailing maintenance schedules, performed actions, and observations for future reference.
- *Temperature and humidity checks:* Regular monitoring of environmental conditions with adjustments must be done as needed to maintain stability.
- *Microbial culture tests:* Conduct random microbial tests of incubators and work platforms to ensure contamination-free environments.
- *Bench tops:* Daily cleaning with distilled water and lab detergent, followed by VOC-free disinfectants, and alcohol cleaning during prolonged breaks.
- *Heating blocks:* Weekly cleaning with distilled water and 70% ethanol; calibrate every 3 months or as needed
- *Pipette handling systems:* Daily sterilization, washing with distilled water, and using lab disinfectants for cleaning
- *Incubators:* Clean and replace water weekly in the water pan. Change gas filters every 6 months and clean monthly with distilled water or 70% ethanol with restabilization periods.
- *CO_2 incubators:* Use autodecontamination programs and ensure medical-grade CO_2 with a 0.22-micron filter.
- *Culture media:* Use commercially available presterilized media properly labeled with batch numbers, manufacture, and expiry dates.
- *Other laboratory equipment:* Keep all equipment clean and sterile with proper storage and handling protocols.
- *Refrigerator:* Use a frost-free refrigerator for media and solutions, ensuring regular temperature monitoring and surface disinfection.
- *Binocular microscope:* Regular cleaning of the microscope stage and focusing knobs, maintaining ambient temperature to prevent fungal growth
- *Centrifuge:* Place on a vibration-free surface, regularly check for vibrations, and perform maintenance as required.
- *Laminar air flow:* Daily cleaning with an alcoholic disinfectant, keeping the cabinet empty except for essential items

Liquid Nitrogen Storage Tanks

Handling and safety precautions for liquid nitrogen (LN_2) are as follows:

- *Protective clothing:* Use cryoprotective gear such as gloves, shoes, and goggles to protect against burns from LN_2.
- *Disease transmission risk:* Vaccination for staff against Hepatitis B to mitigate the risk of disease transmission.

- *Ventilation:* Ensure adequate ventilation in storage areas with oxygen deficiency alarms installed.
- *Daily level checks:* Check and document LN_2 levels daily with alarm systems for low levels.
- *Transport safety:* Use closed and transport Dewars with proper handling protocols to prevent spills and injuries.
- *Maintenance and logbooks:* Maintain detailed maintenance records, decontaminate tanks regularly, and avoid overfilling.
- *General safety protocols:* Train staff on safe handling of LN_2 and emergency procedures and conduct regular safety audits and risk assessments.

STAFFING AND TRAINING

Roles and Responsibilities of Laboratory Personnel

- *Reproductive endocrinologists:* Oversee patient treatment plans and perform clinical procedures.[5]
- *Embryologists:* Handle gamete and embryo manipulation, including IVF, ICSI, embryo culture, and cryopreservation.[6]
- *Andrologists:* Conduct semen analysis and sperm preparation.[8]
- *Anesthesiologists are* competent for short and long procedures.
- *Nurses* assist with procedures and ensure patient comfort.[5]
- *Councilors are* professional individual for counseling the patient on various aspects.
- *Lab technicians* assist with laboratory procedures, equipment maintenance, and data management.[7]
- *Helping staff is* required for helping to shift patient, handle disposal system, and convey messages across various IVF sections.

Training Requirements: Ongoing training and education are essential to keep laboratory personnel updated with the latest advancements. Quality assurance programs include regular internal and external audits to ensure compliance with standards and continuous improvement.[4]

REGULATORY AND SAFETY REQUIREMENTS

Compliance with Local and International Regulations

Assisted reproductive technology laboratories must adhere to a range of regulatory requirements to ensure patient safety and procedural integrity:

- *Licensing and accreditation:* Comply with local health department regulations and obtain necessary licenses and accreditations from recognized bodies
- *Standard operating procedures (SOPs):* Develop and adhere to SOPs for all laboratory processes, ensuring consistency and compliance with regulatory standards.[4]

Safety Protocols and Procedures

Ensuring safety in the ART laboratory involves implementing comprehensive protocols:

- *Personal protective equipment (PPE):* Use gloves, lab coats, and eye protection to prevent exposure to biological and chemical hazards.[4]
- *Emergency procedures:* Well-documented emergency response plans for situations such as chemical spills, fire, and equipment failure are essential.[2]
- *Waste disposal:* Proper disposal methods for biological, chemical, and sharps waste to prevent contamination and injury should be used.[3]

CONCLUSION

Setting up an ART laboratory requires meticulous planning and adherence to strict standards. From designing an efficient layout and equipping the lab with state-of-the-art tools to ensuring staff competency and regulatory compliance, every aspect is crucial for successful and safe ART practices.

REFERENCES

1. Gosden R, Balen AH, Homburg R. Reproductive Medicine: Challenges, Solutions, and Breakthroughs. Cambridge, England: Cambridge University Press; 2013.
2. Mortimer ST, Mortimer D. Quality and risk management in the IVF laboratory. Reproductive Biomedicine Online. 2005;11(5):541-7.
3. European Society of Human Reproduction and Embryology (ESHRE). Guidelines for good practice in IVF laboratories. Hum Reprod. 2010;25(4):798-805.
4. Centers for Disease Control and Prevention (CDC). (2021). Laboratory biosafety manual. [online]. Available from https://www.cdc.gov.tw/Uploads/files/201504/09baa733-ed3b-4531-9753-3841f7c7011a.pdf [Last accessed November, 2024].
5. Carr JJ, Brown JM. Introduction to Biomedical Equipment Technology. London, UK: Pearson; 2013.
6. Nagy ZP, Varghese AC, Agarwal A. Practical manual of in vitro fertilization: Advanced methods and Novel Devices. Berlin, Germany: Springer; 2018.
7. Gardner DK, Weissman A, Howles CM, Shoham Z. Textbook of Assisted Reproductive Techniques: Laboratory perspectives. Boca Raton: CRC Press; 2018.
8. Mortimer D. Practical laboratory andrology. Oxford, UK: Oxford University Press; 2000.
9. Kirkegaard K, Agerholm IE, Ingerslev HJ. Time-lapse monitoring as a tool for clinical embryo assessment. Hum Reprod. 2015;30(8):1813-20.
10. Hardarson T, Van Landuyt L, Jones G. The blastocyst. In: Textbook of Clinical Embryology. Cambridge, England: Cambridge University Press; 2012. pp. 134-45.
11. Fahy GM, Wowk B, Wu J, Paynter S. Improved vitrification solutions based on the predictability of vitrification solution toxicity. Cryobiology. 2004;48(1):22-35.

3 CHAPTER

Quality Control in Assisted Reproductive Technology Laboratory

INTRODUCTION

Quality control (QC) in an assisted reproductive technology (ART) laboratory is paramount for ensuring successful clinical outcomes and maintaining high standards of patient care. QC encompasses a range of procedures and protocols designed to ensure that all laboratory practices and equipment function optimally. This chapter explores the essential components of QC in an ART laboratory, including the importance of QC, standard protocols, and best practices for maintaining the integrity and efficacy of reproductive technologies.

IMPORTANCE OF QUALITY CONTROL

The role of QC in ART laboratories cannot be overstated. The primary goal of ART is to assist individuals in achieving pregnancy, and any deviation from optimal laboratory conditions can significantly impact success rates. High standards of QC ensure that the procedures involved, from gamete handling to embryo culture, are performed consistently and accurately. This consistency is crucial for minimizing risks, preventing contamination, and improving overall success rates.[1]

KEY COMPONENTS OF QUALITY CONTROL

The key components of quality control are:

- *Environmental monitoring:* Environmental monitoring is a critical aspect of QC in an ART laboratory. Factors such as temperature, humidity, air quality, and light exposure can significantly affect the viability of gametes and embryos **(Fig. 1)**. Continuous monitoring systems are employed to ensure these parameters remain within optimal ranges. For instance, incubators should maintain a stable temperature of 37°C and an appropriate level of CO_2 to mimic the human body environment.[2]
- *Equipment maintenance and calibration:* Regular maintenance and calibration of laboratory equipment are essential to ensure accuracy and reliability. Microscopes, incubators, and centrifuges must be routinely checked and serviced. Calibration of equipment should be performed according to the manufacturer's guidelines, and records of maintenance activities should be meticulously kept **(Table 1)**. This ensures that equipment operates correctly and reduces the risk of technical errors during critical procedures.[3]
- *Media and reagents:* The quality of culture media and reagents used in ART procedures directly influences the outcomes. QC protocols must include rigorous testing of media batches for endotoxins, pH levels, and osmolality. Additionally, all reagents should be sourced from reputable suppliers, and their storage conditions must adhere to

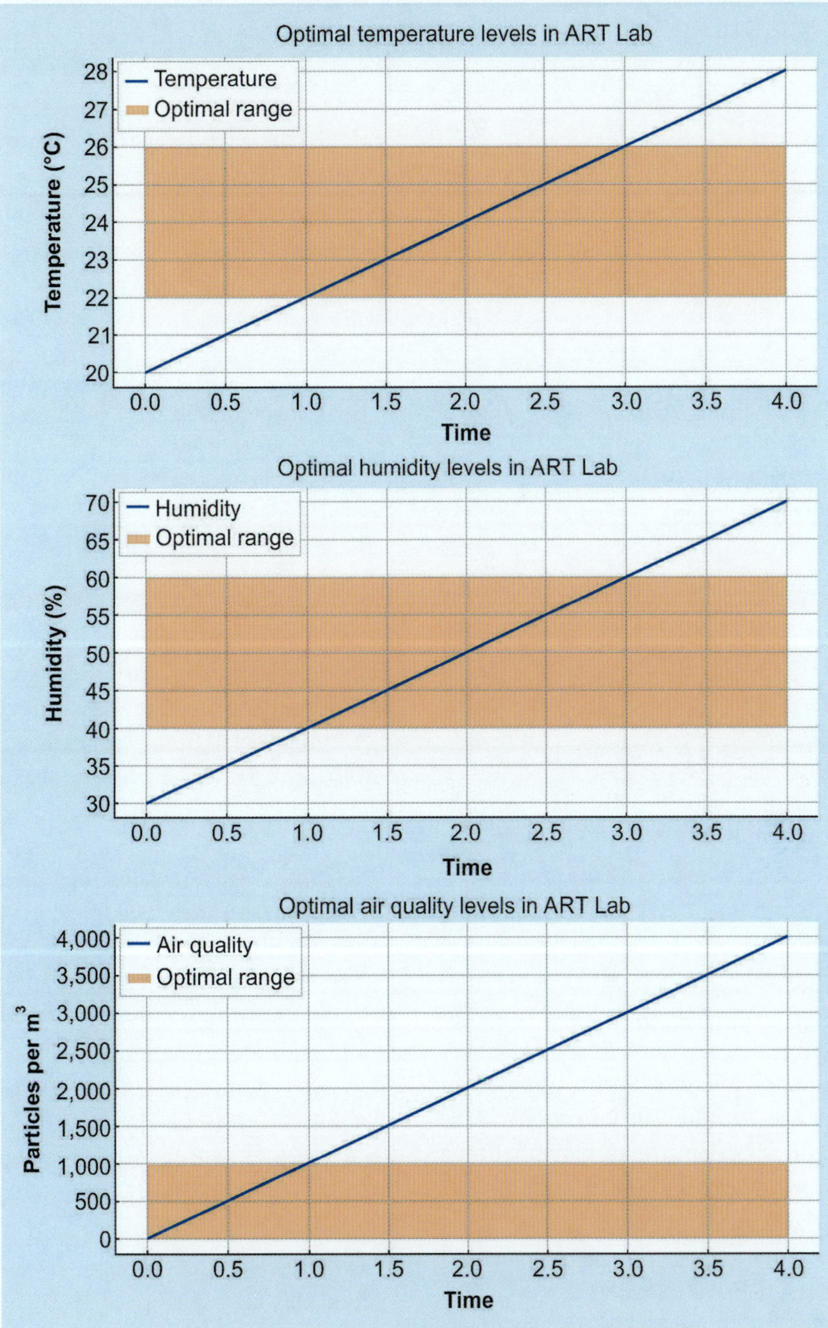

Fig. 1: Environmental conditions in in vitro fertilization (IVF) Lab: Optimum temperature, air quality, and humidity at any given point of time.

TABLE 1: Quality control parameters and frequency for laboratory equipment in assisted reproductive technology (ART).

Equipment	*QC parameter*	*Frequency of QC*
Incubators	Temperature, CO_2/O_2 levels, and humidity	Daily
Laminar flow hood	Airflow velocity and HEPA filter integrity	Monthly
Microscopes (inverted, stereo-zoom)	Optical clarity, alignment, and cleanliness	Weekly
Centrifuges	Temperature control, rotor balance, and RPM accuracy	Weekly
CO_2 analyzers	Calibration and accuracy of CO_2 levels	Monthly
Autoclaves	Sterilization effectiveness and temperature	Monthly
Freezers (cryopreservation units)	Temperature stability and alarm function	Daily
pH meters	Calibration and accuracy of pH measurements	Daily
Gas cylinders	Gas purity and pressure levels	Weekly
Sterilizers	Sterilization cycle validation and spore testing	Monthly
Stereomicroscopes	Focus accuracy and lighting	Weekly
Pipettes	Calibration and volume accuracy	Monthly
Heating stage	Temperature accuracy and uniformity	Daily
Vibration-free tables	Vibration levels	Quarterly
Air quality monitors	Particulate count and VOC levels	Weekly

(HEPA: high-efficiency particulate air; QC: quality control; RPM: revolutions per minute; VOC: volatile organic compounds)

specified requirements to maintain their efficacy.[4]

- *Laboratory personnel:* The competence and training of laboratory personnel are vital components of QC. Staff should undergo regular training sessions and proficiency assessments to ensure they are updated on the latest techniques and protocols. This continuous education helps minimize human error and maintains a high standard of laboratory practice.[5]

PROTOCOLS AND BEST PRACTICES

The protocols and best practices include:

- *Standard Operating Procedures (SOPs):* The development and implementation of SOPs are fundamental to QC in ART laboratories. SOPs provide detailed instructions for every procedure, ensuring consistency and reliability. These documents should be regularly reviewed and updated to incorporate new advancements in ART and regulatory changes.[6]
- *Quality management systems (QMS):* A robust QMS integrates all aspects of QC into a cohesive framework. QMS includes document control, process validation, internal audits, and corrective actions. Implementing a QMS ensures that all laboratory practices are aligned with industry standards and regulatory requirements, thereby enhancing the overall quality of services provided.[7]
- *Regular audits and inspections:* Regular internal and external audits are crucial

for maintaining QC standards. Audits help identify areas of noncompliance and provide opportunities for continuous improvement. External inspections by regulatory bodies ensure that the laboratory meets national and international standards, which is essential for accreditation and certification.[8]

CHALLENGES AND SOLUTIONS

While implementing QC in ART laboratories is essential, it is not without challenges. Common issues include resource limitations, resistance to change, and maintaining consistent standards across all staff members. Solutions to these challenges include:

- Investing in automated monitoring and documentation systems to reduce manual errors and enhance efficiency
- Encouraging a culture of continuous improvement and openness to new technologies and methodologies
- Providing regular training and incentives to staff to maintain high levels of competence and motivation[1]

CONCLUSION

Quality control in an ART laboratory is a multifaceted approach that requires meticulous attention to detail and a commitment to continuous improvement. By implementing comprehensive QC protocols, laboratories can ensure the highest standards of care, thereby maximizing the chances of successful reproductive outcomes. The integration of advanced technologies, regular training, and adherence to SOPs and QMS will pave the way for excellence in ART practices.

REFERENCES

1. Gardner DK, Lane M. Culture systems: The path to improving IVF outcomes. Reprod Biomed Online. 2013; 27(5):505-19.
2. Balaban B, Brison D, Calderón G, Catt J, Conaghan J, Cowan L, et al.; Alpha Scientists in Reproductive Medicine and ESHRE Special Interest Group of Embryology. The Istanbul consensus workshop on embryo assessment: Proceedings of an expert meeting. Hum Reprod. 2011;26(6):1270-83.
3. Mortimer D, Mortimer ST. Quality and Risk Management in the IVF Laboratory. Cambridge, UK: Cambridge University Press; 2005.
4. Hassold T, Hunt P. To err (meiotically) is human: The genesis of human aneuploidy. Nat Rev Genet. 2001;2(4):280-91.
5. Ombelet W, Cooke I, Dyer S, Serour G, Devroey P. Infertility and the provision of infertility medical services in developing countries. Hum Reprod Update. 2008;14(6):605-21.
6. Harper JC, Coonen E, Handyside AH, Winston RM, Delhanty JD. Quality control in the PGD laboratory. Prenatal Diagnosis. 2012;32(4):251-9.
7. Cummins JM. Vigilance and validation: Essentials of QC in the ART laboratory. Fertil Steril. 2013;99(1):47-52.
8. Barton LA, Yazdani A, Taylor TH, Reijnders P. Quality management and accreditation systems in ART laboratories. Reprod Biomed Online. 2014;28(2):134-41.

4 CHAPTER

Semen Analysis According to World Health Organization 2021 Guidelines

INTRODUCTION

Semen analysis is a cornerstone of male fertility evaluation and plays a critical role in understanding reproductive health. The World Health Organization (WHO) 2021 guidelines set the global standard for semen analysis, emphasizing accuracy and consistency in assessing key parameters such as volume, pH, concentration, motility, and morphology. These guidelines provide a structured framework for the proper collection, handling, and examination of semen samples to minimize variability and ensure reliable results. By adhering to these protocols, laboratories can diagnose male infertility with precision, identify potential underlying issues, and guide effective clinical interventions. This chapter explores the essential aspects of semen analysis as outlined in the WHO 2021 manual, offering insights into both basic and advanced assessment techniques.

SAMPLE COLLECTION AND HANDLING

Guidelines for Sample Collection

The World Health Organization (WHO) 2021 guidelines provide comprehensive instructions to ensure the accurate collection of semen samples, which is crucial for reliable analysis. Key considerations include:

- *Abstinence period:* To minimize variability in semen analysis results, the sample should be collected after a minimum of 48 hours but not longer than 7 days of sexual abstinence. Abstinence shorter than 48 hours may lead to lower semen volume and higher sperm concentration, affecting motility assessment. Conversely, abstinence longer than 7 days can increase semen volume and dilute the sperm count, leading to errors in sperm concentration measurements.[1]
- *Collection method:* Masturbation is the preferred method for obtaining a semen sample as it avoids contamination that can occur with other techniques such as coitus interruptus or using latex condoms. The sample should be collected in a wide-mouthed, nontoxic, sterile container designated for single use.[1]
- *Environment:* Samples should ideally be collected in a private room close to the laboratory to ensure the sample's integrity. The collection room should be equipped with necessary supplies such as liquid soap, sterile saline, and disposable containers arranged in a tray for convenience. If collection is done at home, the sample must be delivered to the laboratory within 1 hour, maintaining body temperature by keeping it close to the body.[1]
- *Handling and transportation:* Proper handling is crucial for maintaining sample integrity. After collection, the semen should be kept at body temperature

(37°C). If transportation is necessary, the sample should be protected from extreme temperatures (below 20°C or above 40°C). Accurate labeling with the patient's name, date, time of collection, and duration of abstinence is essential to prevent mix-ups and ensure traceability.[1]

SEMEN PARAMETERS AND ASSESSMENT

Volume, pH, Concentration, Motility, and Morphology

Semen analysis involves evaluating several key parameters **(Table 1)**:

- *Volume:* The volume of semen is measured using a micropipette. Normal ejaculate volume ranges between 1.5 and 7.6 mL. Deviations from this range may indicate issues with seminal vesicle function or ejaculation.[1]
- *pH:* Normal semen pH ranges from 7.2 to 8.0. Abnormal pH levels may indicate infections or issues with the seminal vesicles or prostate. For instance, a pH <7 in azoospermic samples may suggest ejaculatory duct obstruction.[1]
- *Sperm concentration:* A normal sperm concentration is at least 15 million sperm per mL. Lower concentrations (oligozoospermia) can be linked to various infertility issues and require further investigation.[1]
- *Motility:* Sperm motility is categorized into grades (A, B, C, and D) based on movement quality. At least 40% of sperm should exhibit motility, with at least 32% showing progressive motility. This assessment is performed at 37°C using a warmed stage and phase contrast microscopy at 400X magnification.[1]
- *Morphology:* Sperm morphology is assessed by the percentage of sperm with normal forms. A normal sample should have at least 4% normal forms according to strict criteria. Abnormalities in head, neck, midpiece, or tail can significantly impact fertility.[1]

TABLE 1: Lower reference limits for semen characteristics.

Semen characteristic	***Lower reference limit***
Volume, mL	1.4
Sperm concentration, 10^6/mL	16
Total sperm number, 10^6	39
Total motility (PR + NP), %	42
PR, %	30
Vitality (live spermatozoa), %	58
Sperm morphology (normal forms), %	4
pH	≥7.2
Seminal fructose, µmol/ejaculate	≥13

(PR: progressive motility; NP: nonprogressive motility)

Initial Macroscopic Examination

The initial macroscopic examination involves:

- *Liquefaction:* Normal semen liquefies within 15 minutes at room temperature and within 10 minutes at 37°C. Delayed liquefaction should be recorded as it indicates increased viscosity, which can interfere with further analysis.[1]
- *Appearance:* Immediately after liquefaction, the semen should be inspected for homogeneity and color. Normal semen is gray-opalescent. Deviations such as red-brown or yellow hues may indicate blood presence, jaundice, or infection.[1]
- *Viscosity:* Viscosity is assessed by the ease with which semen drops from a pipette. Normal samples form small, discrete drops. High-viscosity samples

form threads longer than 2 cm, affecting motility and concentration assessments.[1]

- *pH measurement:* A drop of semen is spread on pH paper and compared to a calibration strip. Abnormal pH values can indicate ejaculatory duct obstruction or other conditions.[1]

Microscopic Examination

The microscopic examination involves:

- *Sperm concentration:* Using a Neubauer chamber, the sperm concentration is calculated by counting the sperm in specific grid squares after appropriate dilution. If the concentration is very low, a direct count on a slide can be done.[1]
- *Motility assessment:* Sperm motility is categorized into grades, with grade IV indicating rapid linear motility and grade I indicating nonmotile sperm. A systematic count in several fields helps determine the motility percentage, crucial for diagnosing conditions like asthenozoospermia.[1]
    - *Grade IV motility:* Rapid linear motility (i.e., >25 μm/s at room temperature (25 μm is approximately equal to five head lengths or half tail length. In spermatozoa of this grade, tail is not visible as it goes relatively fast and linear.
    - *Grade III:* Slow or sluggish but progressively motile spermatozoa
    - *Grade II:* Nonprogressively motile spermatozoa
    - *Grade I:* Nonmotile spermatozoa
    - *Cellular elements other than spermatozoa:* The presence of cells such as leukocytes, epithelial cells, and immature germ cells is noted. High leukocyte counts may indicate infection and poor sperm quality.[1]
    - *Agglutination and aggregation:* Agglutination, where motile sperm stick together, can indicate the presence of antisperm antibodies. Aggregation refers to the adherence of immotile sperm to mucus, cells, or debris, affecting motility.[1]

Secondary Microscopic Examination

The secondary microscopic examination involves:

- *Sperm vitality:* Sperm vitality is assessed using dye exclusion tests with live sperm remaining unstained. This assessment helps verify motility results and identify structural defects in sperm.[1]
    - *Methods:* Eosin-nigrosin staining, Papanicolaou staining, Diff-Quick reagent staining, hypo-osmotic swelling (HOS) test
    - At least 100 spermatozoa are to be counted with differentiation of live (unstained) and dead (stained). The count is expressed in terms of percentage.
- *Morphology:* Morphological assessment considers abnormalities in the sperm head, neck, midpiece, and tail **(Table 2)**. Specific abnormalities can indicate underlying genetic or exposure issues impacting fertility potential.[1]

Since recommended morphological assessment considers the functional regions of spermatozoon, following are categories of abnormalities **(Fig. 1)**:

- *Head:* Namely large, small, tapered, pyriform, round, amorphous, vacuolated, small acrosomal region, double head, or any combination of these
- *Neck:* Bent and asymmetrical insertion of midpiece into the head
- *Midpiece:* Thick or thin, irregular, or any combination of these; thin midpiece is a characteristic of no mitochondrial sheath

TABLE 2: Standard dimensions and key features of sperm-cell components.

Sperm part	***Description***	***Typical dimensions***
Head	Contains the nucleus and acrosome	• *Length:* 4.0–5.5 µm • *Width:* 2.5–3.5 µm
Acrosome	Cap-like structure covering the anterior part of the head; contains enzymes for penetrating the egg	Covers 40–70% of the head's surface
Midpiece	The section connecting the head to the tail; contains mitochondria for energy	• *Length:* 5.0–7.5 µm • *Diameter:* ~1.0 µm
Tail (flagellum)	Propels the sperm forward, essential for motility	*Length:* 45–55 µm
Nucleus	Located in the head, contains the genetic material (DNA)	Occupies the majority of the head space

(DNA: deoxyribonucleic acid)

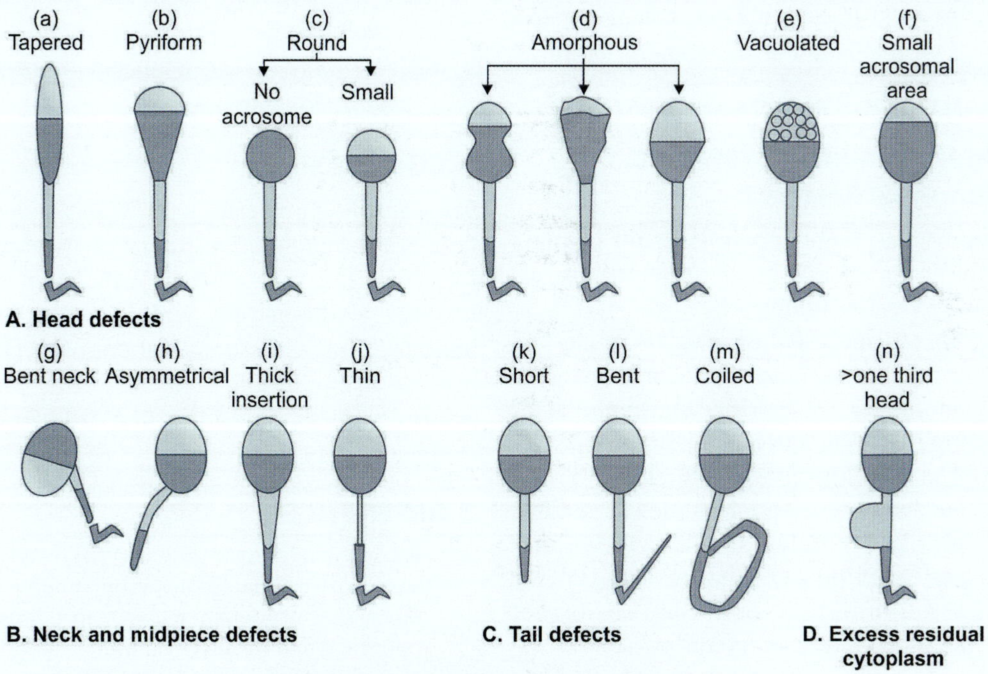

Fig. 1: Various sperm morphology defects.
Source: World Health Organization. 2021.

- *Tail:* Short, multiple, hairpin, broken, bent, irregular width, coiled, or any combination of these
- *Cytoplasmic droplet:* Normally located in the midpiece region, the presence of cytoplasmic droplets can indicate an issue with sperm maturation. Excessive droplets can impair sperm motility and function.

Advanced Tests: Deoxyribonucleic Acid Fragmentation and Oxidative Stress

Advanced tests provide additional insights into sperm quality and fertility potential:

- *DNA fragmentation:* DNA fragmentation tests measure the percentage of sperm with fragmented DNA. High levels of DNA fragmentation can be associated with infertility, miscarriage, and poor assisted reproductive technology (ART) outcomes.[2]
- *Oxidative stress:* Oxidative stress tests assess the balance between reactive oxygen species (ROS) and antioxidants in semen. Elevated ROS levels can damage sperm DNA and membranes, impairing fertility.[3]

INTERPRETATION OF RESULTS

Understanding Normal and Abnormal Results

Interpreting semen analysis results involves comparing measured parameters against WHO reference values:

- *Normal results:* Indicate that the sample falls within the reference range for all assessed parameters, suggesting that male factor infertility is unlikely to be a primary issue.[1]
- *Abnormal results:* Indicate potential fertility issues. Abnormalities in volume, pH, concentration, motility, or morphology each point to different underlying conditions that may require further investigation or intervention.[1]

Clinical Significance of Various Semen Parameters

Each semen parameter provides specific insights into male reproductive health:

- *Volume:* Low ejaculate volume (<1.5 mL) may indicate issues with the seminal vesicles, partial ejaculatory duct obstruction, or retrograde ejaculation.[1]
- *pH:* Abnormal pH can signal infections or problems with the seminal vesicles or prostate. Low pH (<7.2) may be associated with blockages in the ejaculatory ducts.[1]
- *Sperm concentration:* Low sperm concentration (oligozoospermia) is often linked to genetic factors, testicular dysfunction, or hormonal imbalances. It can significantly impact fertility.[1]
- *Motility:* Reduced motility (asthenozoospermia) affects the sperm's ability to reach and fertilize the egg. Causes may include varicocele, infections, or lifestyle factors.[1]
- *Morphology:* Abnormal morphology (teratozoospermia) can result from genetic defects, exposure to toxins, or oxidative stress. It is a significant predictor of fertilization potential.[1]

CONCLUSION

Semen analysis according to WHO 2021 guidelines is a comprehensive evaluation essential for diagnosing male infertility. By adhering to strict guidelines for sample collection, handling, and assessment, laboratories can provide accurate and reliable results that inform clinical decisions and treatment strategies.

REFERENCES

1. World Health Organization (WHO). WHO laboratory manual for the examination and processing of human semen, 6th edition. Geneva: World Health Organization; 2021.
2. Simon L, Emery BR, Carrell DT. Review: Diagnosis and impact of sperm DNA alterations in assisted reproduction. Best Pract Res Clin Obstet Gynaecol. 2017;44:38-6.
3. Agarwal A, Majzoub A, Esteves SC, Ko E, Ramasamy R, Zini A. Clinical utility of sperm DNA fragmentation testing: Practice recommendations based on clinical scenarios. Trans Androl Urol. 2016;5(6):935-50.

5 CHAPTER

Sperm Preparation and Cryopreservation

INTRODUCTION

Sperm preparation and cryopreservation are critical components of assisted reproductive technology (ART), aimed at optimizing sperm quality for successful fertilization and preserving fertility for future use. Techniques such as swim-up, density gradient centrifugation, and advanced methods like microfluidics and magnetic-activated cell sorting (MACS) enable the selection of highly motile, morphologically normal sperm, essential for procedures like IUI, IVF, and ICSI. Cryopreservation, involving freezing and storing sperm at ultra-low temperatures, provides a reliable option for individuals undergoing medical treatments or preserving fertility for later use. Together, these processes enhance fertilization potential and expand reproductive options, making them indispensable in modern ART.

PURPOSE AND METHODS

Objectives of Sperm Preparation

The primary objective of sperm preparation in assisted reproductive technology (ART) is to isolate and enhance the most motile and morphologically normal spermatozoa from a semen sample. This process is crucial for optimizing fertilization rates in procedures such as intrauterine insemination (IUI), in vitro fertilization (IVF), and intracytoplasmic sperm injection (ICSI).[1] Sperm preparation techniques aim to:

- *Remove seminal plasma:* Seminal plasma contains factors that can inhibit sperm function and survival. Removing it is essential to avoid these negative effects.[2]
- *Isolate highly motile sperm:* By selecting sperm with the best motility, the chances of successful fertilization are increased.[3]
- *Eliminate immature and abnormal sperm:* This reduces the presence of sperm with deoxyribonucleic acid (DNA) damage or structural defects, improving the likelihood of selecting sperm capable of successful fertilization and development.[4]

Common Techniques: Swim-up and Density Gradient Centrifugation

Several techniques are commonly employed to prepare sperm for ART procedures **(Table 1)**. Two of the most widely used methods are the swim-up technique and density gradient centrifugation:

- *Swim-up technique:* This method relies on the natural motility of sperm. A semen sample is overlaid with culture medium and motile sperm swim-up into the medium. After a period of incubation, the top layer, which contains the motile sperm, is carefully collected. This technique is simple and effective but may result in lower yield and is more suitable for samples with a high initial sperm concentration.[5]
- *Density gradient centrifugation:* This technique involves layering a semen

TABLE 1: Sperm preparation and cryopreservation medium with their components.

Media type	*Description*	*Components*
Sperm washing media	Used to wash and clean sperm samples to remove debris, dead sperm, and seminal plasma	• Buffered saline solution (e.g., HEPES and MOPS) • Protein supplements (e.g., serum albumin) • Antibiotics
Sperm swim-up media	Used for selecting motile sperm by allowing them to swim-up into a clean medium	• Balanced salt solution (e.g., HTF and PBS) • Protein supplements (e.g., serum albumin)
Density gradient media	Used for separating sperm based on density to isolate the healthiest and most motile sperm	• Silica particles (e.g., Percoll and Sil-Select) • Buffered saline solution and protein supplements
Capacitation media	Used to induce capacitation, a process that enhances sperm's ability to fertilize an egg	• Balanced salt solution • Bicarbonate • Calcium chloride • Protein supplements (e.g., serum albumin)
Cryopreservation media	Used for freezing and storing sperm samples at ultra-low temperatures	• Cryoprotectants (e.g., glycerol, ethylene glycol) • Buffered saline solution • Protein supplements
Sperm activation media	Used to activate sperm motility and prepare them for fertilization	• Balanced salt solution • Calcium chloride • Protein supplements (e.g., serum albumin)

[HEPES: N-hydroxyethylpiperazine-N-ethane sulfonic acid; HTF: human tubal fluid; MOPS: 3-(N-morpholino) propane sulfonic acid; PBS: phosphate-buffered saline]

sample over a gradient of solutions with different densities, typically made from silica-based media. The sample is then centrifuged, causing sperm to migrate through the gradient based on their density. Highly motile, morphologically normal sperm are collected from the bottom layer. This method is highly effective in separating sperm from debris, dead sperm, and seminal plasma, making it suitable for samples with a wide range of qualities.[2]

Additionally, four basic approaches to sperm preparation include:

- *Washing:* It is the oldest technique aimed at removing seminal plasma only. It is simple and quick but does not enrich motile sperm or remove debris effectively.
- *Swim-up from pellet:* It is a widely-used technique based on the active migration of motile sperm into an overlaid medium. It is highly effective in separating motile sperm from nonmotile sperm and debris.

- *Swim-up from ejaculate (overlay method):* It is similar to the swim-up from pellet but avoids centrifugation. It is suitable only for samples with high initial motility.

Advanced Sperm Preparation Techniques

The advanced sperm preparation techniques are:

- *Microfluidics:* It is a cutting-edge technique that uses microfluidic channels to isolate motile sperm based on their swimming ability. This method is highly efficient, reduces the risk of DNA fragmentation, and mimics natural sperm selection processes.
- *Magnetic activated cell sorting (MACS):* It is a method that uses magnetic beads to selectively remove apoptotic (dead or dying) sperm, enhancing the quality of the sample by increasing the proportion of viable sperm.
- *Zeta potential selection:* This technique relies on the natural charge differences between healthy and damaged sperm to selectively enrich for viable, motile sperm.
- *Fertile chip (microfluidic sperm sorting):* It is a specialized microfluidic chip that isolates the healthiest sperm by simulating the natural reproductive process, ensuring that only the best sperms are selected for use.

OPTIMIZATION OF SPERM PREPARATION

Enhancing Sperm Quality and Function

Optimizing sperm preparation involves several strategies to enhance the quality and functionality of the selected sperm:

- *Antioxidant treatments:* Adding antioxidants to sperm preparation media can reduce oxidative stress, thereby improving sperm motility and DNA integrity. This can be particularly beneficial for samples with high levels of reactive oxygen species (ROS).[2]
- *Temperature control:* Maintaining samples at a consistent, optimal temperature (37°C) throughout the preparation process is crucial for preserving sperm motility and viability.[6]
- *Optimal timing:* Timing the incubation and centrifugation steps precisely is essential. Over-incubation can lead to a decline in sperm motility and viability, while inadequate incubation may result in insufficient separation of motile sperm.[5]

Troubleshooting Common Issues

Addressing common issues in sperm preparation is vital for achieving the best possible outcomes:

- *Low sperm yield:* If the yield of motile sperm is low, adjusting the centrifugation speed and duration or using a different gradient density may help improve recovery. Ensuring proper technique in layering the gradients and careful aspiration of the sperm layer are also critical.[2]
- *Poor sperm motility:* Poor motility may be addressed by optimizing the composition of the preparation media, including the use of motility enhancers or specific buffers that support sperm function. Ensuring that the sample is processed quickly and at optimal temperatures can also help maintain motility.[6]
- *High levels of debris:* High levels of cellular debris can be minimized by careful initial semen handling and pretreatment with simple washes before applying the main preparation technique. Using a two-layer density gradient instead of a single layer can also enhance separation.[3]

SEMEN CRYOPRESERVATION

Cryopreservation is a method used to preserve cell viability over extended periods by maintaining them at extremely low temperatures. The primary aim of any cryopreservation protocol is to minimize damage to cell membranes caused by exposure to low temperatures, control cell volume, and prevent the formation of lethal intracellular ice crystals.[2] Achieving these objectives involves controlling molecular movement both inside and outside the cell. The principle of semen cryopreservation is to sustain sperm viability by cooling and storing them in liquid nitrogen at approximately -196°C. This process requires the addition of a cryopreservation medium.

When a cryoprotectant is added, sperm cells undergo rapid shrinkage as intracellular water exits the cell in response to the hyperosmotic extracellular solution. Gradually, the cell returns to its original volume as the cryoprotectant permeates the cell. The presence of cryoprotective agents in both intracellular and extracellular fluids lowers the freezing point, allowing the solutes to remain in their actual freezing state. Ice formation starts in the extracellular medium, and as water molecules leave to form ice crystals, the freezing point of the remaining solution continuously drops, increasing extracellular osmotic pressure. This draws more intracellular water out, dehydrating the cell and reducing the risk of lethal intracellular ice formation.[2]

Cryodamage mechanisms include the loss of superoxide dismutase enzyme from the plasma membrane, loss of acrosomal integrity, and increased plasma membrane permeability. These cell-altering events are associated with the cryopreservation and thawing processes.[6]

Cryopreservation Protocol

Cryopreservation protocol involves the following:

- *Labeling:* Cryovials are precisely labeled with patient-specific details and unique identity codes to ensure accurate tracking and identification. All essential information is thoroughly recorded in both a physical logbook and digital records, maintaining robust documentation and traceability.
- *Preparation:* Bring both the preservation medium and semen sample to room temperature.
- *Mixing:* Add the preservation medium to the semen sample in a 1:1 ratio, adding the medium drop-by-drop with gentle stirring to ensure thorough mixing.
- *Filling vials:* Fill cryo vials with the mixture, label them with identifying information, and date them.
- *Initial cooling:* Place the vials at the neck of the cryo cane (a relatively warmer region) for 30 minutes.
- *Prefreezing:* Move the vials to the level of the liquid nitrogen for an additional 30 minutes.
- *Freezing:* Submerge the vials in liquid nitrogen for long-term storage.
- *Thawing:* Begin by carefully identifying and confirming that the freezing code matches the logbook records. Once verified, remove the cryovial from the liquid nitrogen and allow it to thaw at room temperature. After the sample has fully liquefied, typically within about 10 minutes, proceed with the subsequent procedures.

Benefits of cryopreserving semen:

- *Extended fertility options:* It allows for the possibility of conception at a much later date.

- *Preservation of healthy sperm:* It preserves sperm that are normal and healthy for future use when only abnormal or no sperm might be present.
- *Optimal timing for insemination:* It enables sperm to be used for insemination under optimal conditions without the need for a fresh sample at that specific time.[2]

Applications

Patients who might benefit from sperm cryopreservation include those undergoing medical treatments that could impair sperm production or transport, such as surgery, radiation therapy, chemotherapy, or other interventions affecting ejaculatory function. It is also useful during vasectomy reversals as a precaution against possible subsequent blockage of the vas deferens and during testicular, epididymal, or vas biopsies, especially in cases of azoospermia. Additionally, it helps in cases of highly variable semen quality or quantity and when the male partner is unavailable during optimal insemination times.[5]

Men undergoing treatment for tumors that require surgical removal of the testis, radiation to the groin, or chemotherapy often utilize cryopreservation to ensure future fertility options. In cases of oligozoospermia (low sperm count), several vials of concentrated sperm can be pooled at the time of insemination to increase the chances of pregnancy.

Demerits

Demerits of cryopreservation are as follows:

- *Uncertain pregnancy outcomes:* There is no guarantee that cryopreserved and subsequently thawed sperm will lead to pregnancy.
- *Equipment failure:* Technical failures can occur, although alarms and backup systems are in place to minimize the risk.
- *Reduced sperm quality:* Cryopreservation and thawing often reduce sperm viability and motility. For some men, the process can result in most or all sperm becoming nonmotile or dead.
- *Infection risks:* There is a risk of transmitting infections present in the semen at the time of cryopreservation, similar to the risks associated with using fresh semen.[6]

Despite these challenges, semen cryopreservation remains a valuable technique in ART, providing significant benefits for fertility preservation and assisted conception.

CONCLUSION

Sperm preparation and cryopreservation are integral components of ART that demand precision and a thorough understanding of the underlying biological processes. By adhering to established protocols and continuously refining techniques, ART laboratories can significantly enhance the quality and viability of sperm used in reproductive procedures. The integration of cutting-edge methodologies, procedural adherence, and ongoing evaluation of outcomes will ensure that sperm preparation and preservation contribute effectively to the success of ART, ultimately improving the likelihood of positive reproductive outcomes.

REFERENCES

1. Agarwal A, Majzoub A, Esteves SC, Ko E, Ramasamy R, Zini A. Clinical utility of sperm DNA fragmentation testing: Practice recommendations based on clinical scenarios. Transl Androl Urol. 2016;5(6): 935-50.
2. Esteves SC, Varghese AC, Agarwal A. A concise review of the relevance of time

lapse imaging in human sperm retrieval and selection. Clinics. 2015;70(8):567-71.
3. Mortimer D. Practical laboratory andrology. Oxford, UK: Oxford University Press; 2000.
4. Parmegiani L, Cognigni GE, Bernardi S, Troilo E, Ciampaglia W, Filicori M. Physiologic ICSI: Hyaluronic acid (HA) favors selection of spermatozoa without DNA fragmentation and with normal nucleus, resulting in improvement of embryo quality. Fertil Steril. 2010;93(2):598-604.
5. Sakkas D, Ramalingam M, Garrido N, Barratt CL. Sperm selection in natural conception: What can we learn from mother nature to improve assisted reproduction outcomes? Hum Reprod Update. 2015;21(6): 711-26.
6. Simon L, Lewis SEM. Sperm DNA damage or DNA fragmentation: the predictive value for successful outcomes in assisted reproduction. Human Reprod. 2011;26(7):1921-31.

6 CHAPTER

Culture Systems and Media

INTRODUCTION

Culture systems and media are essential in assisted reproductive technology (ART), providing the optimal environment for oocyte and embryo development by supplying necessary nutrients, energy sources, and growth factors while maintaining critical conditions like pH, temperature, and osmolarity. Different media types, such as sequential, single-step, and synthetic formulations, address the unique needs of embryos at various stages, ensuring their development. Advanced innovations like dynamic culture systems, time-lapse imaging, and microfluidics further refine the process, enhancing embryo viability, implantation success, and overall outcomes in fertility treatments.

TYPES OF CULTURE MEDIA

Composition and Purpose of Different Media Types

Culture media are essential for the in vitro development of embryos in assisted reproductive technology (ART). These media provide the necessary nutrients, energy sources, and environmental conditions that support the growth and development of oocytes and embryos.

- *Basic culture media:* These media are designed to provide the fundamental components required for cell survival and initial development. They typically contain salts, glucose, amino acids, vitamins, and bicarbonate for pH buffering. Examples include human tubal fluid (HTF) and Krebs–Ringer bicarbonate solution (KSOM).[1]
- *Sequential media:* These are specialized media used at different stages of embryo development. Early cleavage-stage embryos have different nutritional requirements compared to blastocysts **(Table 1)**. Sequential media systems, such as G1 and G2 media, are designed to mimic these changing needs. G1 media support the early cleavage stages, while G2 media are formulated for the blastocyst stage.[2]
- *Single-step media:* Unlike sequential media, single-step media are formulated to support embryo development from fertilization to the blastocyst stage without the need to change the media. This approach minimizes embryo handling and stress. Examples include global and continuous single culture (CSC) media.[3]
- *Synthetic oviductal fluid (SOF):* This media is designed to mimic the fluid found in the oviduct and uterus, providing an environment that closely resembles the in vivo conditions. SOF media contain a mix of amino acids, vitamins, and energy substrates suitable for both cleavage and blastocyst stages.[4]

Commercially available culture media offer a diverse range of options, each

TABLE 1: Key requirements of embryos during pre-compaction and post-compaction stages.

Stage	*Pre-compaction (cleavage stage)*	*Post-compaction (blastocyst stage)*
Developmental focus	Rapid cell division and formation of the morula	Cell differentiation and blastocoel cavity formation
Energy requirements	Primarily pyruvate and lactate for energy	Increased glucose uptake for energy
Nutritional needs	Amino acids, minimal glucose, and low oxygen concentration	Complex mix of amino acids, higher glucose, and oxygen levels
Environmental needs	Low oxygen tension (5–7%), controlled pH, and temperature	Slightly higher oxygen tension, stable pH, and optimal temperature
Growth factors	Basic growth factors (e.g., TGF-β, EGF) supporting early cell proliferation	Enhanced growth factors (e.g., IGF, FGF) promoting cell differentiation
Metabolic activity	Lower metabolic activity focusing on initial cleavage divisions	Increased metabolic activity to support blastocyst expansion and differentiation
Morphological changes	Initial cell division, formation of blastomeres	Formation of trophectoderm and inner cell mass
Osmolarity	Lower osmolarity to support blastomere formation	Slightly higher osmolarity to maintain blastocoel integrity
pH requirements	Tight pH control around 7.2–7.4	More tolerant to pH variations, but optimal around 7.3–7.4
Culture media	Pre-compaction media (e.g., early-stage or cleavage-stage media)	Post-compaction media (e.g., blastocyst or advanced-stage media)

(EGF: epidermal growth factor; FGF: fibroblast growth factor; IGF: insulin-like growth factor; TGF-β: transforming growth factor beta)

designed to meet the specific needs of embryo development. These media often include pH indicators to monitor and ensure the integrity of the cold chain, providing a reliable measure of quality throughout the storage and handling process.

Sequential Media

Sequential media are formulated to meet the specific nutritional and environmental needs of embryos at different stages of development. Early-stage embryos and blastocysts have distinct requirements, and sequential media systems are designed to accommodate these differences.

- *Early embryo development media:* This support early cleavage-stage embryos by providing the necessary components to ensure proper cell division and growth.
- *Advance stage embryo development media:* Tailored for the later stages, particularly the blastocyst stage, this media contain nutrients that support the embryo's continued development and differentiation.

The application of sequential media is crucial in optimizing the conditions for each developmental stage, ultimately improving the chances of successful implantation and pregnancy **(Table 2)**.

TABLE 2: Comparative features between sequential media and single-step media used in assisted reproductive technology (ART) laboratories.

Feature	*Sequential media*	*Single-step media*
Nutrient composition	Staged nutrient composition for each embryo development stage	Uniform nutrient composition throughout the development process
Usage process	Requires multiple media changes during different embryo development stages	Uses a single medium for the entire culture period
Time efficiency	Requires more handling and time for media changes	More time-efficient due to reduced handling
Embryo development stages	Different media tailored for specific development stages (e.g., cleavage, blastocyst)	One medium supports all stages of embryo development
Success rates	Historically used with proven success rates	Increasingly popular with comparable or better success rates

Single-step Media

Single-step media are designed to provide a continuous environment for embryo development, eliminating the need for media changes. This approach reduces the handling of embryos, thereby minimizing stress and potential damage.

- *Universal embryo culture media:* This is a widely used single-step media that support all stages of embryo development, from fertilization to the blastocyst stage
- *CSC media:* Another example of single-step media, CSC media is formulated to maintain a stable environment throughout the embryo's development, enhancing the likelihood of successful outcomes.

Single-step media are particularly beneficial in laboratories where minimizing embryo manipulation is a priority, as they allow for a simplified and streamlined culture process.

Custom Media Formulations

In addition to commercially available options, some laboratories opt to use custom formulations tailored to specific needs. Custom media formulations allow ART practitioners to optimize the components and conditions to better suit their patient populations or to incorporate the latest research findings.[3]

- *Tailored nutrient composition:* Custom formulations can adjust nutrient levels to address specific patient needs or improve embryo quality based on recent scientific insights.
- *Incorporation of new additives:* New additives, such as antioxidants or growth factors, can be included in custom formulations to enhance embryo development and improve outcomes.

CULTURE SYSTEMS

Culture systems are designed to provide the optimal environment for embryo development, and they can be broadly classified into static and dynamic systems.

- *Static culture systems:* These are the traditional systems where embryos are cultured in a stationary droplet of media under mineral oil. This setup is simple and cost-effective, allowing for easy monitoring and manipulation of embryos. However, static systems do not mimic the dynamic conditions of the in vivo environment.[5]

- *Dynamic culture systems:* These systems aim to better replicate the physiological conditions by introducing movement and fluid flow. Examples include microfluidic devices and rotating wall vessel bioreactors. Microfluidic systems provide a controlled flow of media around the embryos, mimicking the natural transport of nutrients and waste. Rotating wall vessel bioreactors create a gentle, continuous movement that prevents embryos from settling and simulates the dynamic uterine environment.[6]

Oil and Oil Overlay

Oil overlay is a vital technique in embryo culture systems, where a layer of oil, typically mineral or paraffin oil, is placed over the culture medium. This method is essential for maintaining the stability of the culture environment **(Table 3)**. The oil overlay prevents the evaporation of the culture medium, ensuring that osmolarity and pH levels remain stable, which are crucial for proper embryo development.

Additionally, the oil acts as a protective barrier, shielding the culture from potential contaminants like dust and microorganisms, and helping to maintain a sterile environment. It also provides thermal insulation, helping to keep the culture at the required temperature. By using an oil overlay, the consistency and reliability of the embryo culture conditions are significantly enhanced, which is crucial for the success of ARTs.

Media for Handling and Preparation of Oocytes and Sperms

Hyaluronidase (Hydase)

- *Purpose:* Hyaluronidase is an enzyme-based medium used to remove the cumulus cells surrounding the oocyte after retrieval **(Table 4)**. These cells are bound together by hyaluronic acid, and the enzyme hyaluronidase breaks down this substance, allowing the cumulus cells to be gently removed.

TABLE 3: Overview of oil types and their characteristics in in vitro fertilization (IVF).

Type of oil	*Description*
Mineral oil	A purified oil derived from petroleum, often used in IVF due to its stability and inert properties; it maintains stability even when subjected to temperature variations during the cooling chain. Typically used as is due to its inert nature
Paraffin oil	A highly refined oil with lower viscosity, derived from hydrocarbons; it is known for its clarity and purity. It stays stable under cold storage conditions, ensuring its properties remain intact during transportation and storage. It is often mixed with pressure oil to enhance media compatibility
High-viscosity oil	It is an oil with higher viscosity, providing better insulation and reducing the risk of medium evaporation
Silicone oil	It is a synthetic oil known for its high stability and low reactivity, offering excellent thermal properties
Low-viscosity oil	It is a more fluid oil that spreads easily over the culture medium, providing quick coverage and ease of use

TABLE 4: Hyaluronidase variants for effective oocyte denudation in in vitro fertilization (IVF).

Type of hyaluronidase	*Concentration*	*Description*
Hyaluronidase 80 IU/mL	80 IU/mL	Standard concentration for routine oocyte denudation procedures
Hyaluronidase 100 IU/mL	100 IU/mL	Higher concentration for more efficient cumulus cell removal
Hyaluronidase 150 IU/mL	150 IU/mL	Enhanced enzyme activity for rapid denudation in specific cases
Hyaluronidase 200 IU/mL	200 IU/mL	High concentration for challenging cases requiring quick action

TABLE 5: Polyvinylpyrrolidone (PVP) variants for optimal sperm handling in in vitro fertilization (IVF).

Types of PVP	*Description*
PVP 7%	Commonly used concentration for routine sperm immobilization during intracytoplasmic sperm injection (ICSI)
PVP 10%	Higher viscosity for more precise sperm selection and handling
PVP 12%	Used for cases requiring enhanced control over sperm movement
PVP 15%	Provides maximum viscosity for difficult sperm manipulation

- *Application:* Essential in the denudation process, hyaluronidase ensures that the oocyte is prepared for fertilization, particularly in procedures like intracytoplasmic sperm injection (ICSI), where a clear view of the oocyte is necessary.

Polyvinylpyrrolidone

- *Purpose:* Polyvinylpyrrolidone (PVP) is a synthetic polymer used in sperm preparation, particularly in ICSI. It acts as a viscous medium to slow down the movement of sperm, making it easier to select and immobilize individual sperm for injection into the oocyte **(Table 5)**.
- *Application:* PVP is crucial for handling and manipulating sperm during ICSI, ensuring that only the most viable sperm are selected and reducing the risk of damage to the oocyte during the injection process.

Advances in Culture Technologies

Recent advances in culture technologies have significantly improved the success rates of ART procedures. Some of the notable innovations include:

- *Time-lapse imaging:* This technology allows for continuous monitoring of embryo development without disturbing the culture conditions. Time-lapse systems like the embryoscope provide detailed images of embryos, enabling better assessment and selection based on developmental milestones.[7]
- *Microfluidics:* These devices use small volumes of fluids to create a more physiologically relevant environment for embryos. Microfluidic systems can precisely control the microenvironment, reduce the stress on embryos, and improve nutrient delivery.[8]
- *3D culture systems:* Traditional 2D culture methods may not fully replicate the 3D structure of the in vivo environment. 3D culture systems use scaffolds or gels

to provide a more realistic architecture, enhancing cell interactions and developmental potential.[9]

- *Artificial intelligence (AI):* AI and machine learning algorithms are being developed to analyze time-lapse images and predict embryo viability more accurately than traditional methods. These technologies can enhance the selection process, leading to higher implantation and pregnancy rates.[10]

CONCLUSION

The choice and optimization of culture media in an ART laboratory are vital to ensuring the best possible environment for embryo development. By carefully selecting the right media—whether it is sequential, single-step, or custom formulations, laboratories can significantly boost the chances of successful outcomes. It is a process that requires attention to detail, a willingness to adapt, and a commitment to using the latest advancements. By doing so, ART practices can achieve higher success rates and provide better care for patients, ultimately leading to more successful reproductive outcomes.

REFERENCES

1. Biggers JD, Summers MC, McGinnis LK. Polyvinyl alcohol and amino acids as substitutes for bovine serum albumin in culture media for mouse preimplantation embryos. Hum Reprod Update. 2005;11(3):169-75.
2. Gardner DK, Lane M. Culture and selection of viable blastocysts: a feasible proposition for human IVF? Hum Reprod Update. 1998;4(4):431-46.
3. Sunde A, Brison D, Dumoulin J, Harper J, Lundin K, Magli MC, et al. Time to take human embryo culture seriously. Hum Reprod. 2016;31(10):2174-82.
4. Tervit HR, Whittingham DG, Rowson LE. Successful culture in vitro of sheep and cattle ova. J Reprod Fertil. 1972;30(3):493-7.
5. Swain JE. Optimizing the culture environment in the IVF laboratory: impact of pH and buffer capacity on gamete and embryo quality. Reprod Biomed Online. 2014;28(5):484-90.
6. Wheeler MB, Walters EM, Clark SG. Advances in the production of transgenic livestock. Transgenic Research. 2006;15(6):673-86.
7. Kirkegaard K, Agerholm IE, Ingerslev HJ. Clinical use of time-lapse imaging in embryo selection: a systematic review. Human Reproduction Update. 2012;18(4):613-24.
8. Zheng W, Xie Y, Zhang H, Zhang X, Wang D. A microfluidics approach to the study of human embryonic stem cell pluripotency. Lab on a Chip. 2012;12(8):1233-44.
9. Hickman DL, Rigas JD, Hughes C, Lackford B, Gierahn TM, Rothenberg EV. 3D tissue models: a new frontier in biomaterials research. Biomaterials. 2014;35(24):6047-56.
10. VerMilyea M, Hall JMM, Diakiw SM, Johnston A, Nguyen T, Perugini D, et al. Development of an artificial intelligence-based assessment model for prediction of embryo viability using static images captured by optical light microscopy during IVF. Hum Reprod. 2020;35(4):770-84.

CHAPTER 7

Oocyte Retrieval

INTRODUCTION

Oocytes are typically retrieved 36 hours after the administration of human chorionic gonadotropin (hCG), agonist or antagonist, triggering luteinizing hormone (LH) surge and utilizing ultrasonography for guidance. The follicular aspirates are then examined under a stereo zoom microscope equipped with a transmitted illumination base and a heated stage. The contents of each tube are distributed into 2–3 Petri dishes to create a thin fluid layer, allowing for a careful and efficient search for oocyte–cumulus complex (OCC) within the follicular tissue.

The appearance of the oocyte can vary depending on its maturity. It is often surrounded by cumulus cells, and a highly mature oocyte, which may appear pale and be difficult to identify. Granulosa cells are more transparent and "fluffy", appearing in amorphous, often-iridescent clumps. Blood clots from the collection needle should be carefully dissected using 23-gauge needles to check for cumulus cells. Once identified, the OCC should be promptly transferred to the appropriate culture environment for in vitro fertilization (IVF). The oocytes are maintained in 5% CO_2 at 37°C until the semen is prepared for insemination. If the oocytes appear immature, they are incubated for an additional 4–6 hours to achieve maturation before insemination.

- Oocytes that are luteinized may appear very pale and difficult to locate, with the cumulus cells breaking down into a gelatinous mass around the oocyte, resulting in a lower probability of fertilization.
- Atretic oocytes exhibit granulosa cells with a lace-like appearance and are typically dark and hard to identify.
- Dysmorphic oocytes can be identified by cytoplasmic granularity, areas of necrosis, organelle clustering, vacuolization, and anomalies of the zona pellucida. These oocytes have a reduced potential for implantation and development, often resulting in biochemical pregnancies.[1]

Nuclear maturity is a critical factor in assessing oocyte quality, significantly influenced by the oocyte's environment. LH plays a central role in the maturation process necessary for completing the first meiotic division. Elevated LH levels can indicate premature oocyte maturation, leading to physiological aging and decreased fertilization potential.[1]

OOCYTE MATURATION

Current ovarian stimulation regimens often produce follicles of varying sizes, leading to a lack of synchronization in development. Oocyte maturation involves a complex sequence of intracellular changes, including nuclear and cytoplasmic maturation. A mature oocyte ready for fertilization should be in metaphase II stage. There is no direct correlation between follicle size and oocyte

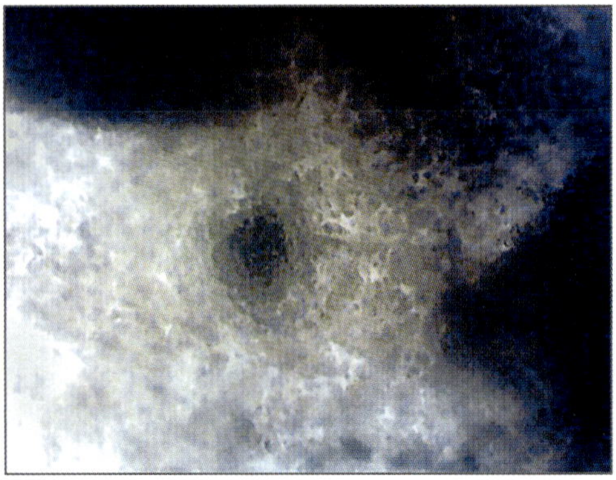

Fig. 1: Immature oocyte–cumulus complex (OCC) with tightly packed cumulus cells.

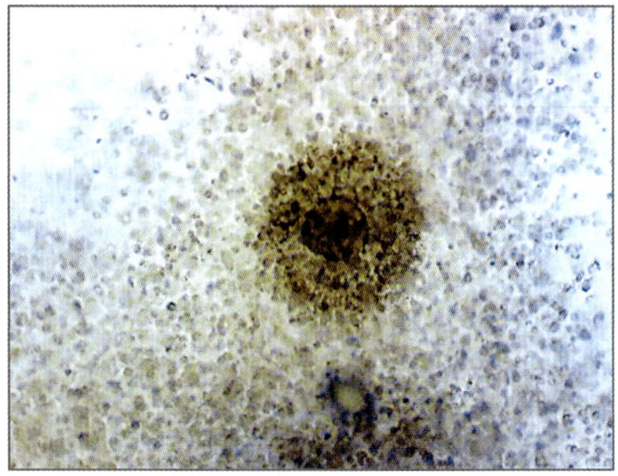

Fig. 2: Mature oocyte–cumulus complex (OCC) with sunburst-like appearance of cumulus cells.

maturity, which is why all aspirated oocytes are typically incubated in a culture medium for 2–3 hours at 37°C in 5% CO_2 before insemination.[2]

OOCYTE–CUMULUS COMPLEX GRADING

Once identified, oocytes are graded based on the expansion of the cumulus mass and the compactness of the corona cells surrounding them:

- *Grade 1:* Immature oocyte with no germinal vesicle breakdown; corona cells are tightly packed, appearing as a dark ring with scanty cumulus cells **(Fig. 1)**.
- *Grade 2:* Germinal vesicle breakdown has occurred, but there is no extrusion of the first polar body (metaphase I). Corona cells remain tightly packed, forming a dark ring, and cumulus cells are also tightly packed.
- *Grade 3:* Mature oocyte with the first polar body extruded (metaphase II); corona cells are less tightly packed, forming a lighter ring, and cumulus cells are loosened and abundant.
- *Grade 4:* Mature oocyte, usually preovulatory (metaphase II); corona cells appear "sunburst", and cumulus cells are fully expanded and abundant **(Fig. 2)**.
- *Postmature:* The oocyte is dark in appearance, with gelatinous or mucified cumulus cells and degenerating corona cells **(Fig. 3)**.[3]

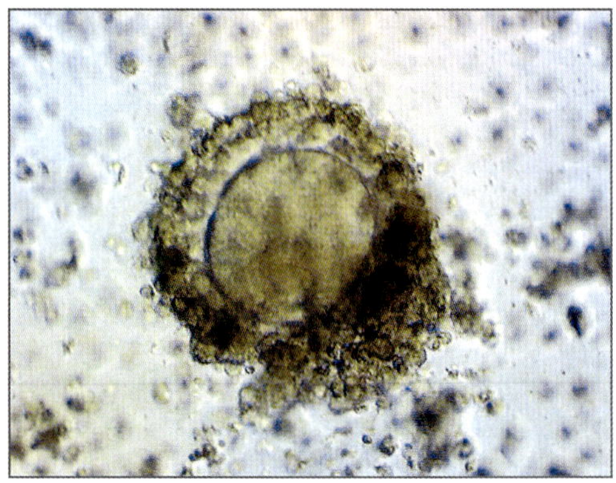

Fig. 3: Postmature oocyte–cumulus complex (OCC) with dispersed cumulus cells.

CONCLUSION

The process of oocyte retrieval is fundamental to the success of IVF. The timing, handling, and assessment of the oocytes are critical factors that directly influence the outcomes of the procedure. By ensuring that the oocytes are retrieved at the optimal stage of maturity and maintained in an environment conducive to their development, the chances of successful fertilization and subsequent embryo development are significantly enhanced. The grading of oocytes based on their cumulus complex and morphological characteristics further aids in selecting those with the highest potential for successful implantation, thus, optimizing the overall success rates of assisted reproductive technologies.

REFERENCES

1. Veeck LL. Oocyte assessment and biological performance. Ann N Y Acad Sci. 1988;541(1): 259-74.
2. Edwards RG. Follicular fluid. J Reprod Fertil. 1974;37(1): 189-219.
3. Eppig JJ. Coordination of nuclear and cytoplasmic oocyte maturation in eutherian mammals. Reprod Fertil Dev. 1996;8(4): 485-9.

CHAPTER 8

In Vitro Fertilization

INTRODUCTION

In vitro fertilization (IVF) is a fundamental procedure in assisted reproductive technology (ART), enabling the fertilization of oocytes outside the human body under controlled conditions. The process involves key steps such as oocyte insemination, fertilization assessment, and embryo development, each designed to maximize the likelihood of a successful outcome. Oocytes are exposed to motile sperm, followed by careful evaluation to identify signs of fertilization, including pronuclei formation and cytoplasmic changes. Techniques like cumulus denudation and zygote grading are used to select the most viable oocytes and embryos for further development. IVF has transformed the landscape of reproductive medicine, providing hope to individuals and couples dealing with infertility and paving the way for ongoing advancements in treatment and success rates.

INSEMINATION (IN VITRO FERTILIZATION)

During the insemination process, oocytes are typically exposed to a concentration of 100,000 motile sperm per milliliter. If the prepared sperm demonstrates suboptimal motility or morphology, the concentration may be increased accordingly.[1] Each washed oocyte is transferred into a droplet containing motile sperm at the specified concentration **(Table 1)**. A quick check under an inverted microscope ensures that the oocytes are neither over- nor under-inseminated.[2] The inseminated oocytes are then incubated in a CO_2 incubator at 37°C for 16–20 hours.[3]

TABLE 1: Insemination guidelines based on oocyte–cumulus complex (OCC) maturation stages.

Oocyte–cumulus complex (OCC) maturation stage	*Insemination type*	*Notes*
Immature OCC	High insemination (30,000–35,000 sperms/OCC)	A higher number of sperm is required to penetrate the tightly packed cumulus cells surrounding immature OCCs
Mature OCC	Standard insemination (20,000–25,000 sperms/OCC)	A balanced number of sperm is used, appropriate for the optimal fertilization potential of mature OCCs, where the cumulus is moderately packed
Post-mature OCC	Low insemination (10,000–15,000 sperms/OCC)	Fewer sperm are required to penetrate the loosely packed cumulus cells surrounding post-mature OCCs

DENUDATION OF CUMULUS

Approximately 16–20 hours postinsemination, the cumulus is removed from each oocyte to check for signs of fertilization, indicated by the presence of two pronuclei (PN). Cumulus removal is performed mechanically using pipette with a diameter slightly larger than that of the oocyte. Gentle suction and release facilitate the cell removal process. Care must be taken to avoid damaging the zona pellucida or the oocyte by puncturing or excessive distortion.[4] After removing the cumulus, each oocyte is transferred to a fresh culture droplet under light mineral oil or paraffin oil.[5]

FERTILIZATION OF OOCYTES

Fertilization assessment typically occurs 18–22 hours postinsemination under an inverted microscope to ensure accurate scoring. A normally fertilized oocyte should have two PN and two polar bodies, maintaining a regular shape, an intact zona pellucida, and clear, healthy cytoplasm **(Table 2)**. The cytoplasm of a fertilized oocyte often appears granular, forming a cortical zone, unlike the featureless cytoplasm of an unfertilized oocyte.[2] It is crucial to distinguish vacuoles from PN and other cytoplasmic irregularities. Detailed records of the morphology and fertilization status of each zygote are kept for reference during embryo selection.[1]

Sequence of Events

- *Formation of second polar body (PB2):* The extrusion of the PB2 is the first observable sign of successful fertilization. This occurs approximately 1–3 hours after sperm entry into the oocyte.
- *Appearance of 2 PN:* Approximately 16–20 hours postfertilization, the male and female PN become visible. The presence of 2 PN indicates normal fertilization.
- *Alignment of PN and nucleoli:* By 20–22 hours postfertilization, the PN align toward the center of the zygote. The nucleoli within the PN also become organized, often forming a symmetric pattern.

TABLE 2: Guidelines for zygote assessment after in vitro fertilization.

Parameter	*Assessment criteria*
Pronuclei (PN)	1 PN—unipronuclear; 2 PN—normally fertilized; 3 or more PN—polyspermic or abnormal fertilization
Nucleoli (N) in PN	Number and alignment (symmetric or asymmetric) of N within each PN; uniform and aligned N are optimal
Cytoplasmic halo	Presence or absence of a halo around the PN; a clear, well-defined halo is considered optimal
Polar bodies	Number, size, and position of polar bodies; normal zygotes typically have two visible polar bodies
Cytoplasmic appearance	Homogeneity of cytoplasm; homogeneous cytoplasm without visible granularity is considered optimal
Zygote score (Z-score)	Calculated based on the number and position of N, the presence of a halo, and other factors; used to rank zygotes
Time of observation	Typically assessed 16–20 hours postinsemination or intracytoplasmic sperm injection (ICSI)

- *PN migration toward each other:* Between 22 and 24 hours postfertilization, the PN move closer to each other as they prepare for syngamy.
- *Syngamy (fusion of PN):* Syngamy occurs around 24–26 hours postfertilization, where the male and female PN fuse to form a single diploid nucleus. This marks the formation of the zygote.
- *First mitotic division begins:* The zygote begins its first mitotic division approximately 26–30 hours postfertilization.
- *Zygote becomes a two-cell embryo:* By 30–32 hours postfertilization, the zygote completes its first division and becomes a two-cell embryo, marking the beginning of embryonic development.

Grading of fertilization involves assessing and separating abnormally fertilized oocytes for separate culture. Delayed fertilization, with PN appearing on day 2, can result from oocyte or sperm defects, either morphological or endocrine.[3]

During fertilization, over 500 capacitated spermatozoa typically surround the cumulus complex. These sperm must penetrate the cumulus and the zona pellucida to reach the perivitelline space. Simultaneously, the oocytes must prevent additional sperm from entering to avoid polyspermic fertilization. In the perivitelline space, the sperm head binds to the vitelline membrane at the equatorial segment of the acrosome. The sperm head is then taken into the ooplasm through a phagocytic mechanism, forming the male pronucleus. Concurrently, a membrane forms around the female chromosomes, creating the female pronucleus. The fusion of these two PN, known as syngamy, marks the beginning of the zygote's rapid mitotic division process, known as cleavage.[5]

CONCLUSION

The process of in vitro fertilization (IVF) involves a series of timed and carefully controlled steps that are crucial for successful fertilization and subsequent embryonic development. Each stage, from insemination to fertilization assessment, requires precise execution to maximize the chances of achieving a viable pregnancy. The use of advanced techniques, such as the grading of oocytes and zygotes, ensures that only the most promising are selected for further development. As reproductive technology continues to evolve, these practices will likely become even more refined, offering higher success rates and more favorable outcomes for those undergoing assisted reproductive treatments.

REFERENCES

1 Johnson R, Patel S, Kumar A, Smith T, Lee H, Garcia M. Advanced Techniques in Oocyte Insemination. Reproductive Medicine Journal. 2023;38(1):45-6.
2. Smith A, Robinson K, Wong P, Ellis J, Carter M, Zhang Q. Oocyte Retrieval and Insemination Protocols. Journal of Assisted Reproduction and Genetics. 2022;39(5):678-89.
3. Brown C, Taylor E, Scott R, Adams P, Green J, Hughes L. Evaluation of Oocyte Fertilization and Early Embryo Development. Fertility and Sterility. 2020;114(3):421-32.
4. Clark D, Mitchell R, Johnson L, Carter E, Wright P, Torres F. Mechanical Methods for Cumulus Removal in Oocyte Handling. Endocrine Reviews. 2019;40(2):210-22.
5. Jones B, Cooper D, Walker S, Khan L, Reed A, Patel V. Detailed Analysis of Fertilization Processes in Assisted Reproductive Technologies. Reproductive Biology and Endocrinology. 2021;19(1):24-36.

CHAPTER 9

Oocyte Denudation

INTRODUCTION

Oocyte denudation is a crucial step in assisted reproductive technology (ART), particularly in procedures like in vitro fertilization (IVF) and intracytoplasmic sperm injection (ICSI). This process involves the removal of cumulus cells surrounding the oocyte, enabling the evaluation of its maturity and quality while facilitating the precise injection of sperm during ICSI. The timing of denudation, typically 1 to 3 hours post-retrieval, is critical for maintaining oocyte viability and developmental potential. Various techniques, including mechanical and enzymatic methods, are employed to ensure efficient cumulus cell removal while preserving oocyte integrity. Effective denudation improves fertilization outcomes, supports embryonic development, and plays a pivotal role in optimizing ART success rates.

PURPOSE AND TIMING

Importance of oocyte denudation: Oocyte denudation is a critical step in assisted reproductive technology (ART), particularly in the processes of in vitro fertilization (IVF) and intracytoplasmic sperm injection (ICSI). Denudation involves the removal of the cumulus cells surrounding the oocyte, thereby exposing the zona pellucida and enabling the evaluation of oocyte maturity and quality. The cumulus cells play a crucial role during the final stages of oocyte maturation and provide necessary support through paracrine signals. However, the removal of cumulus cells is crucial for ICSI, as it enables the direct injection of sperm into the oocyte.[1] This process also facilitates the precise determination of the sperm injection site, ensuring optimal visualization of the polar body.

The importance of denudation lies in its impact on the fertilization process. Cumulus cells can interfere with the accurate assessment of oocyte morphology, which is essential for selecting the best oocytes for fertilization.[2] Moreover, during ICSI, the presence of cumulus cells can hinder the precise injection of a single spermatozoon into the oocyte. Therefore, effective denudation facilitates better assessment and handling of oocytes, thereby improving fertilization outcomes and subsequent embryonic development.

Optimal Timing Postretrieval

The timing of oocyte denudation is pivotal for ensuring the highest chances of successful fertilization and embryonic development. Typically, oocytes are denuded approximately 1–3 hours postretrieval. This interval allows for the stabilization of the oocyte environment after retrieval from the ovarian follicles, which is beneficial for subsequent handling and manipulation.[3]

Delaying denudation beyond this optimal window can have detrimental effects on oocyte quality. Prolonged exposure of oocytes to in vitro conditions without cumulus cells can lead to cytoplasmic and nuclear maturation discrepancies, negatively affecting the oocyte's developmental potential.[4] Therefore, adhering to the recommended timing is crucial to maintain oocyte viability and enhance ART outcomes.

TECHNIQUES

Mechanical versus Enzymatic Methods

Two primary techniques are employed for oocyte denudation: Mechanical and enzymatic. Each method has its own advantages and limitations, and the choice often depends on the specific requirements of the ART procedure and the preference of the laboratory personnel.

Mechanical methods: Mechanical denudation involves the use of pipettes and repeated pipetting to physically remove cumulus cells. This method is advantageous as it avoids the use of potentially harmful chemicals, thus reducing the risk of oocyte damage. However, it requires skill and precision to avoid physical damage to the oocyte.[5]

Enzymatic methods: Enzymatic denudation utilizes enzymes such as hyaluronidase to digest the hyaluronic acid matrix that binds

TABLE 1: Comparison of group denudation versus individual denudation techniques.

Parameter	***Group denudation***	***Individual denudation***
Technique	Multiple oocyte–cumulus complexes are denuded simultaneously in the same dish	Each oocyte–cumulus complex is denuded separately in its own dish or well
Efficiency	Faster process due to simultaneous handling of multiple oocytes	Slower process as each oocyte is handled individually
Oocyte handling	Requires careful coordination to avoid damage to multiple oocytes during simultaneous denudation	Allows for more precise and controlled handling of each oocyte, reducing the risk of mechanical damage
Cumulus removal	Removal of cumulus cells may be less uniform due to simultaneous processing	More consistent removal of cumulus cells
Time management	More time-efficient for processing large numbers of oocytes	More time-consuming, especially when dealing with a high number of oocytes
Preferred dish setup	Larger dishes or multi-well plates such as four-well dish to accommodate multiple oocytes	Individual droplets or wells to maintain separation and prevent mixing
Potential for oocyte loss	Higher potential for loss of oocytes due to simultaneous processing and handling	Lower potential for loss as each oocyte is handled separately, with more attention to detail
Clinical outcome consideration	Suitable for high-throughput IVF laboratories where time efficiency is critical	Preferred in situations where oocyte quality is paramount, and the risk of damage needs to be minimized
Preferred application	Used in high-volume settings where the time saved can outweigh the risks associated with group handling	Used in settings prioritizing high precision, such as cases with a low number of oocytes

cumulus cells together. This method is efficient and less labour-intensive, allowing for the quick and thorough removal of cumulus cells. However, the use of enzymes necessitates careful control of enzyme concentration and exposure time to prevent potential damage to the oocyte.[6]

BEST PRACTICES FOR SUCCESSFUL DENUDATION

Successful oocyte denudation requires adherence to best practices to ensure the preservation of oocyte quality and viability. Key practices include:

- *Standardized protocols:* Establishing and following standardized protocols for both mechanical and enzymatic denudation helps maintain consistency and minimizes the risk of oocyte damage **(Table 1)**.[7]
- *Training and skill:* Proper training of laboratory personnel in handling and denudation techniques is crucial. Skilled technicians can effectively perform denudation with minimal oocyte trauma, thereby preserving oocyte integrity and developmental potential.[8]
- *Optimal conditions:* Maintaining optimal laboratory conditions, such as temperature and pH, during denudation is essential. This helps preserve the oocyte's microenvironment and enhances the chances of successful fertilization and embryo development.[9]
- *Minimizing exposure time:* Reducing the time oocytes spend outside the incubator and exposed to suboptimal conditions during denudation can significantly impact their quality. Quick yet careful handling ensures that oocytes remain viable and capable of successful fertilization.[10]

CONCLUSION

By adhering to the abovementioned best practices, ART laboratories can optimize the outcomes of oocyte denudation, leading to improved fertilization rates and better overall success in reproductive treatments.

REFERENCES

1. Ménézo Y, Veiga A. Assisted Reproductive Techniques: Challenges and Management Options. Berlin: Springer;2010.
2. Nagy ZP, Gardner DK, Sakkas D, Schoolcraft WB. Clinical Aspects of ICSI. Berlin: Springer; 2005.
3. Van Blerkom J. Epigenetic influences on oocyte developmental competence: periconceptional environment, follicular differentiation, and intrafollicular vascularization. Reproductive BioMedicine Online. 2011;22(6):627-40.
4. Rienzi L, Ubaldi F, Iacobelli M, Ferrero S, Minasi MG, Sapienza F, et al. Embryo culture systems. Reproductive BioMedicine Online. 2012;24(6):634-643.
5. Elder K, Dale B. In-vitro Fertilization. Cambridge: Cambridge University Press; 2010.
6. Sakkas D, Trounson AO. Embryo Physiology and Assessment of Viability. Berlin: Springer; 2010.
7. Magli MC, Gianaroli L, Fortini D, Ferraretti AP, Fiorentino A, Tosti E. Impact of oocyte dysmorphisms on the outcome of assisted reproduction. Reproductive BioMedicine Online. 2008;16(6):720–8.
8. Vanderzwalmen P, Zech H, Birkenfeld A, Schneider M, Stecher A, Vobornik R. Oocyte and Embryo Morphology. Boca Raton: CRC Press; 2012.
9. Wang Q, Sun QY. Evaluation of oocyte quality: morphological, cellular and molecular predictors. Reprod Fertil Dev. 2007;19(1): 1-12.
10. Swain JE, Smith GD. Advances in embryo culture platforms: novel approaches to improve preimplantation embryo development through modifications of the microenvironment. Hum Reprod Update. 2011; 17(5):541-57.

CHAPTER 10

Oocyte Grading

CRITERIA FOR GRADING

Morphological Assessment Criteria

Oocyte grading is a crucial process in assisted reproductive technology (ART). It involves the evaluation of oocyte quality based on specific morphological characteristics **(Table 1)**. These characteristics are critical indicators of the oocyte's potential for successful fertilization and subsequent embryo development.

TABLE 1: Latest classification system: Alpha Scientists in Reproductive Medicine and ESHRE Special Interest Group of Embryology (2011).

Criteria	*Description*
Cumulus–corona complex	Evaluates the expansion and appearance of the cumulus cells surrounding the oocyte
Cytoplasm	Assesses the homogeneity, granularity, and presence of inclusions within the cytoplasm
Polar body	Checks the presence, shape, and fragmentation of the first polar body
Overall morphology	Considers the overall appearance, including any irregularities or abnormalities
Grades	Oocytes are categorized into different grades based on the combination of these criteria, providing a comprehensive assessment of oocyte quality: A (best quality), B, C, D (poorest quality)

(ESHRE: European Society of Human Reproduction and Embryology)

Key morphological assessment criteria include:

- *Cytoplasmic appearance:* The cytoplasm should be homogenous and free of inclusions. Granular cytoplasm or the presence of vacuoles can be indicative of poor oocyte quality.[1]
- *Perivitelline space:* The space between the oocyte membrane and the zona pellucida should be clear and of a regular size. An enlarged or irregular perivitelline space may suggest oocyte maturation issues.[2]
- *Zona pellucida:* This outer layer should be uniform in thickness and free from abnormalities. Irregularities in the zona pellucida can impact sperm binding and penetration.[3]
- *Polar body:* The presence and morphology of the first polar body are critical. An intact and appropriately sized polar body is a marker of oocyte maturity.[4]
- *Cumulus cells:* While not a direct part of the oocyte, the quality and expansion of cumulus cells can also provide indirect information about the oocyte's developmental potential.[5]

Classification Systems and Scoring

Several classification systems have been developed to standardize the grading of oocytes **(Table 2)**. These systems typically

TABLE 2: Oocyte classification system.

Classification system	***Year***	***Criteria***	***Description***
Zamboni[8]	1987	Morphology	It classifies oocytes based on the presence or absence of the germinal vesicle, cytoplasm appearance, and the surrounding cumulus cells
Veeck[9]	1988	Morphology and maturity	It categorizes oocytes into five grades (A to E) based on cytoplasmic and nuclear maturity: Grade A (best quality) to grade E (poorest quality)
Hillensjö et al.[10]	1990	Maturity and appearance	This divides oocytes into three categories: Mature (M), immature (I), and degenerate (D), based on the presence of the first polar body and cytoplasmic characteristics
De Sutter et al.[11]	1996	Polar body and cytoplasm	It classifies oocytes into four categories based on the visibility of the first polar body and cytoplasmic characteristics: Normal, slightly abnormal, moderately abnormal, severely abnormal
Cummins et al.[12]	1999	Cytoplasm and polar body	It uses cytoplasmic inclusions and the presence of the polar body to categorize oocytes into three groups: Normal, moderately abnormal, and severely abnormal
Ebner et al.[4]	2003	Morphology and polar body	This grades oocytes based on cytoplasmic and polar body appearance into four groups (A to D): A (best quality), B, C, D (poorest quality)
Alpha Scientists in Reproductive Medicine and ESHRE Special Interest Group of Embryology	2011	Comprehensive morphology evaluation	The latest system provides a detailed assessment of oocyte quality by evaluating the cumulus–corona complex, cytoplasm, polar body, and overall morphology

(ESHRE: European Society of Human Reproduction and Embryology)

involve scoring oocytes based on the presence and severity of morphological abnormalities. One common system is the Gosden and Lee classification, which categorizes oocytes into four grades based on cytoplasmic and extracytoplasmic attributes:

- *Grade I:* Oocytes with uniform cytoplasm and regular zona pellucida and perivitelline space
- *Grade II:* Minor cytoplasmic granularity or vacuoles but otherwise normal morphology
- *Grade III:* Significant cytoplasmic granularity or irregularities in the zona pellucida
- *Grade IV:* Severe abnormalities in cytoplasm, zona pellucida, or perivitelline space[6]

Another widely used method is the Maturity Grading System, which focuses on the stage of oocyte maturation:

- *Germinal vesicle (GV):* It represents the earliest stage of oocyte maturation, characterized by the presence of a visible nucleus (GV). The oocyte remains arrested in the prophase of the first meiotic division, indicating its immaturity and readiness for further maturation under appropriate conditions **(Fig. 1)**.
- *Metaphase I (MI):* It denotes the transition phase of oocyte maturation, where the oocyte has resumed meiosis and progressed to the first metaphase stage. At this point, the oocyte is undergoing chromosomal alignment, preparing for the completion of the first meiotic division, but it has not yet reached full maturity **(Fig. 2)**.
- *Metaphase II (MII):* It indicates a fully mature oocyte that has completed the first meiotic division and extruded the first polar body **(Table 3)**. This stage is characterized by the alignment of chromosomes on the metaphase plate,

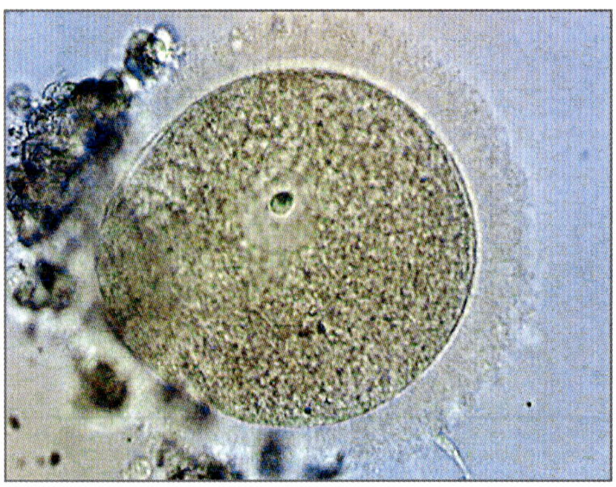

Fig. 1: Germinal vesicle (GV) stage oocyte.

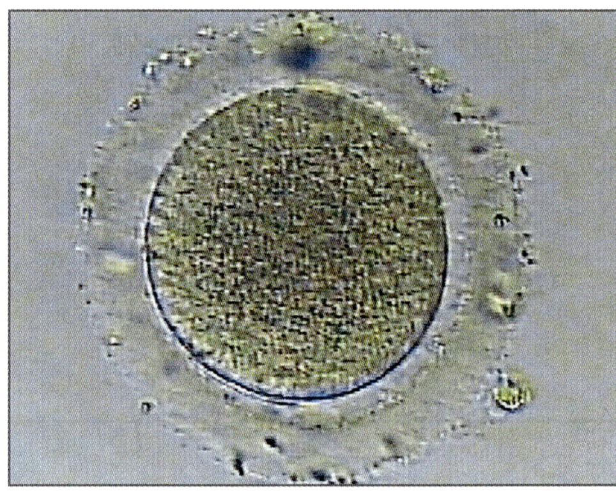

Fig. 2: Metaphase I (MI) stage oocyte.

TABLE 3: Key morphological and biochemical characteristics of a normal human oocyte.

Oocyte characteristic	*Value/range*	*Description*
Oocyte diameter	100–120 µm	The overall size of the human oocyte, including the zona pellucida
Zona pellucida thickness	13–15 µm	The thickness of the outer glycoprotein layer surrounding the oocyte
Perivitelline space	5–10 µm	The space between the zona pellucida and the oocyte membrane
Cytoplasmic granularity	Homogeneous	The cytoplasm of a healthy oocyte is uniformly granular without clumping
First polar body	Intact, smooth surface	Presence of an intact first polar body indicates meiotic competence.
Oocyte membrane integrity	Intact	The oocyte membrane remains intact, ensuring cellular viability

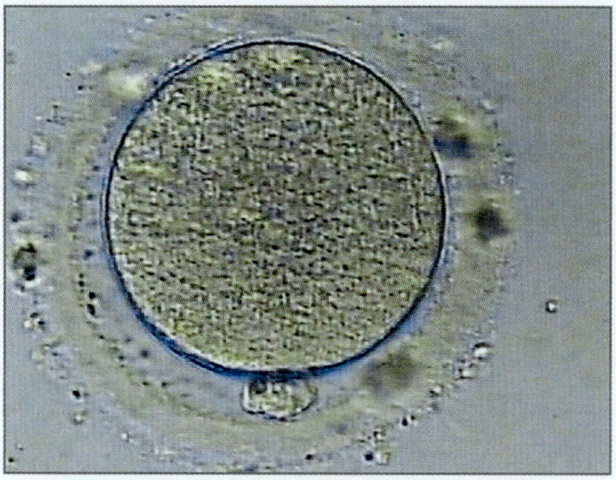

Fig. 3: Metaphase II (MII) stage oocyte.

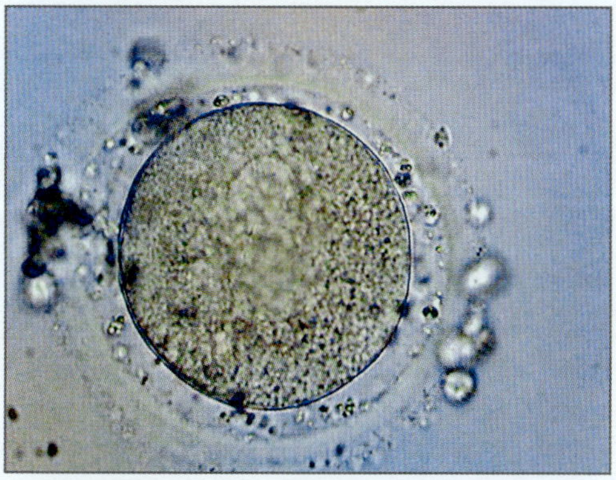

Fig. 4: Oocyte exhibiting multiple vacuoles.

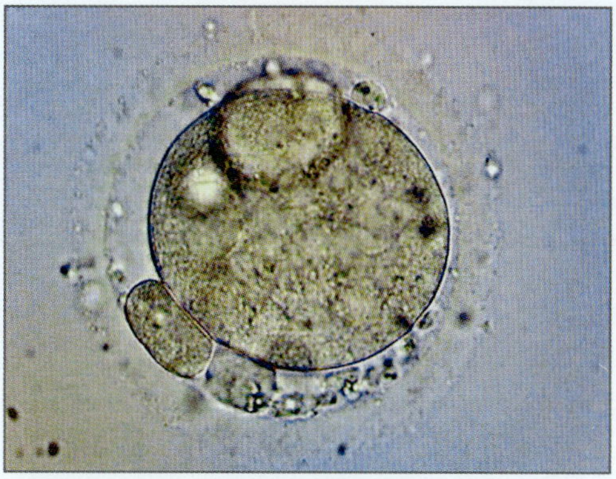

Fig. 5: Oocyte with multiple polar bodies and fragmentation.

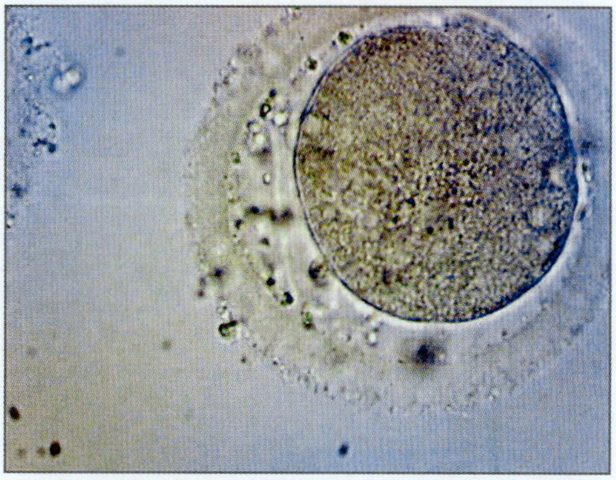

Fig. 6: Oocyte displaying granulation with septate zona.

rendering the oocyte capable of successful fertilization and subsequent embryonic development **(Fig. 3)**.[7]

These systems help embryologists standardize the assessment process, facilitating consistent evaluation and selection of oocytes for fertilization.

CLINICAL RELEVANCE

Correlation Between Oocyte Quality and In Vitro Fertilization Outcomes

The quality of oocytes is directly correlated with the success rates of in vitro fertilization (IVF) treatments. High-quality oocytes are more likely to undergo successful fertilization, develop into healthy embryos, and result in successful pregnancies. Studies have demonstrated that morphological features of oocytes can predict their developmental competence. For example, oocytes with homogeneous cytoplasm and intact polar bodies are associated with higher fertilization rates and better embryo quality.[2]

Conversely, oocytes exhibiting morphological abnormalities often show lower fertilization rates, poor embryo development, and decreased pregnancy outcomes **(Figs. 4 to 7)**. Issues such as cytoplasmic vacuolization, irregular zona pellucida, and

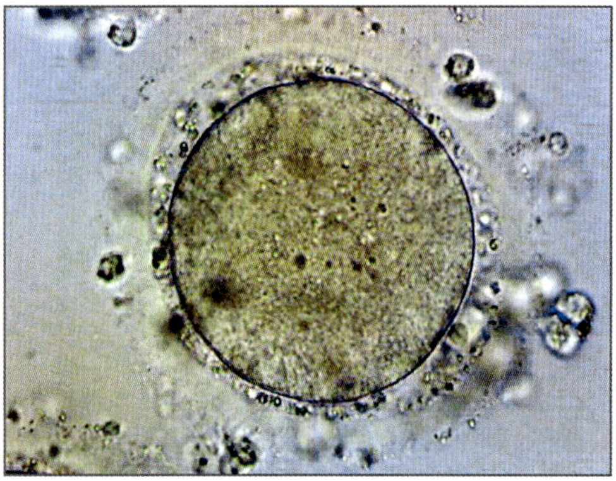

Fig. 7: Oocyte containing perivitelline space debris.

abnormal polar bodies can adversely affect oocyte competence and embryo viability.[4]

Implications for Treatment Planning

Oocyte grading plays a pivotal role in the planning and customization of fertility treatments. By accurately assessing oocyte quality and factors affecting it, clinicians can make informed decisions regarding the best course of action for each patient **(Table 4)**. For instance, patients with predominantly high-quality oocytes may proceed with standard IVF protocols, while those with lower quality oocytes might benefit from additional interventions, such as preimplantation genetic testing or oocyte donation.[5]

Moreover, oocyte grading provides valuable feedback for refining ovarian stimulation protocols. Understanding the relationship between stimulation regimens and oocyte quality can help optimize protocols to enhance the retrieval of high-quality oocytes in future cycles.[3]

CONCLUSION

Grading of oocytes based on morphological criteria is integral to the success of IVF treatments. It enables the selection of the

TABLE 4: Comprehensive overview of biochemical factors influencing oocyte quality.

Factor	*Biochemical impact on oocyte quality*
Age	Mitochondrial dysfunction reduces ATP production, impairing oocyte maturation, fertilization, and early embryonic development
	Increased oxidative stress leads to DNA damage, chromosomal abnormalities, and impaired oocyte quality
Gonadotropins	Excessive FSH stimulation, especially in older women, can cause premature luteinization and reduce oocyte quality
	Abnormal LH levels can disrupt oocyte maturation and ovulation, with elevated LH negatively impacting oocyte quality in polycystic ovary syndrome (PCOS)
Human chorionic gonadotropin (hCG)	Improper timing or dosage of hCG can result in immature oocytes or premature ovulation, affecting oocyte quality
	hCG influences signaling pathways within the oocyte, affecting cell cycle progression and cytoskeletal rearrangements
Pathological conditions	*PCOS:* Hyperandrogenism and insulin resistance lead to impaired folliculogenesis and oocyte quality
	Endometriosis: Inflammatory cytokines and oxidative stress reduce oocyte quality, fertilization rates, and embryo development
Body weight	*Obesity:* Increased adiposity leads to elevated leptin, insulin resistance, chronic inflammation, and impaired oocyte maturation
	Underweight: Low body weight results in hypoestrogenism, anovulation, and the production of poor-quality oocytes

Contd...

Contd...

Factor	*Biochemical impact on oocyte quality*
Smoking	Toxic compounds such as nicotine cause oxidative stress, DNA damage in oocytes, reduced ovarian reserve, and altered follicular fluid
	Smoking accelerates ovarian aging, leading to a decline in oocyte quality and quantity at a younger age
Alcohol consumption	Alcohol increases the production of ROS, causing oxidative damage in oocytes and affecting mitochondrial function crucial for maturation and fertilization
	Chronic alcohol consumption disrupts the hypothalamic–pituitary–ovarian axis, leading to altered levels of gonadotropins and sex steroids, impairing oocyte development and quality
Stress	Chronic stress elevates cortisol levels, disrupting the hypothalamic–pituitary–gonadal axis, leading to impaired oocyte maturation
	Stress-induced oxidative stress can damage oocyte DNA and cellular structures, leading to decreased oocyte quality, fertilization, and embryogenesis

(ATP: adenosine triphosphate; FSH: follicle-stimulating hormone; LH: luteinizing hormone; ROS: reactive oxygen species)

best oocytes for fertilization, improves the predictability of treatment outcomes, and guides personalized treatment strategies to maximize the chances of achieving a successful pregnancy.

REFERENCES

1. Rienzi L, et al. Oocyte morphology predicts outcome of intracytoplasmic sperm injection. Hum Reprod. 2008;23(4):780-6.
2. Balaban B, Urman B. Effect of oocyte morphology on embryo development and implantation. Reprod Biomed Online. 2006;12(5):608-15.
3. Evers JLH. Female subfertility. Lancet. 2013;381(9868):1551-60.
4. Ebner T, et al. Morphological aspects of oocyte maturation and their relevance to preimplantation embryo quality. Reprod Biomed Online. 2003;7(5): 519-29.
5. Mikkelsen AL, Lindenberg S. Morphology of in-vitro matured oocytes: Impact on fertility treatment. Reprod Biomed Online. 2001;3(2):182-4.
6. Gosden RG, Lee B. Classification and grading of oocytes. Assisted Reproductive Technology: Success in a Changing World. Cambridge: Cambridge University Press; 2010. pp. 223-40.
7. Kahraman S, et al. Pronuclear morphology scoring and its impact on embryo development and pregnancy outcome. Reprod Biomed Online. 2000;1(2): 178-83.
8. Zamboni L. Morphology: Classification of oocytes based on the presence or absence of the germinal vesicle, cytoplasmic appearance, and surrounding cumulus cells. 1987.
9. Veeck LL. Morphology and maturity: Categorization of oocytes into five grades (A to E) based on cytoplasmic and nuclear maturity. Ann N Y Acad Sci. 1988;541(1): 259-74.
10. Hillensjö T, Nilsson L, Hamberger L. Maturity and appearance: Division of oocytes into three categories (Mature, Immature, and Degenerate) based on the presence of the first polar body and cytoplasmic characteristics. Hum Reprod. 1990.
11. De Sutter P, Dozortsev D, Qian C, Dhont M. Polar body and cytoplasm: Classification of oocytes into four categories based on the visibility of the first polar body and cytoplasmic characteristics. Hum Reprod. 1996;11(1):173-9.
12. Cummins JM, et al. Oocyte assessment criteria: Evaluating oocyte quality through morphological and cytoplasmic features. Hum Reprod. 1999;14(4):807-15.

11 CHAPTER

Intracytoplasmic Sperm Injection

INTRODUCTION

Intracytoplasmic Sperm Injection (ICSI) has revolutionized the field of assisted reproductive technology, offering hope to patients with severe male infertility. First introduced in 1992 by Palermo and colleagues, ICSI involves the direct injection of a single sperm into an oocyte's cytoplasm, bypassing natural barriers to fertilization. This technique quickly became the cornerstone of in vitro fertilization (IVF) treatments, addressing conditions such as low sperm count, poor motility, and abnormal morphology. Over the years, advancements in micromanipulation tools and laboratory protocols have enhanced the precision and success rates of ICSI. This chapter delves into the evolution of ICSI, its technical intricacies, and its critical role in achieving successful fertilization and embryo development.

The first successful intracytoplasmic sperm injection (ICSI) embryo and pregnancy were reported in 1992 when Palermo and colleagues accidentally injected a human spermatozoon into the ooplasm of a human oocyte during a subzonal sperm injection (SUZI) procedure.[1] Initially, ICSI only marginally improved fertilization outcomes compared to SUZI. Today, ICSI is a highly effective procedure widely used in in vitro fertilization (IVF) laboratories around the world.

Before 1992, severe male infertility cases were often untreatable, leading to a fertilization failure rate of up to 30% in IVF treatments for male infertility. Artificial insemination with donor sperm was the standard treatment. ICSI has revolutionized this field, offering a significant chance for these patients to fertilize oocytes and develop healthy embryos. It is now the first-line treatment for a variety of qualitative or functional sperm disorders.[2]

First-line applications for ICSI:

- IVF fertilization failure
- Sperm agglutination
- Severe oligozoospermia and cryptozoospermia
- Severe asthenozoospermia (e.g., Kartagener syndrome)
- Teratozoospermia, including globozoospermia and pinhead sperm
- Immunological factors such as antisperm antibodies
- Azoospermia, both obstructive and nonobstructive, including cases of paraplegia
- Ejaculatory dysfunction, such as retrograde ejaculation
- Impaired spermatogenesis or spermiogenesis, including immature spermatozoa and various stages of spermatids and spermatocytes
- Oncology patients with cryopreserved sperm before chemotherapy or radiotherapy
- Hepatitis C positive men
- Diagnostic ICSI to evaluate oocyte quality at retrieval

- Rescue ICSI after failed IVF
- Prevention of polyspermy in patients with a history of repeated polyspermy
- Preimplantation genetic diagnosis (PGD)
- In vitro matured oocytes

Intracytoplasmic sperm injection requires the temporary breaching of both the oolemma (egg membrane) and the sperm plasma membrane. Success is indicated by the free flow of ooplasm and permanent immobilization of the sperm tail, making ICSI a technically demanding procedure.[3] ICSI bypasses several upstream events in natural fertilization, such as sperm motility acquisition, capacitation, acrosome reaction, and zona pellucida binding. Instead, a selected and immobilized spermatozoon is directly injected into the cytoplasm of an oocyte after rupturing the oolemma.

PREPARATION AND TECHNIQUE

Preparation for Intracytoplasmic Sperm Injection

Handling of oocytes: Mature oocytes are highly sensitive to environmental changes, particularly deviations in pH and temperature. The type of buffer used in the culture medium and its temperature are therefore critical factors. Even if these conditions do not immediately impact fertilization rates, they can have long-term effects on embryo quality, potentially leading to lower pregnancy rates.[4]

The media used for flushing and aspirating oocytes are typically buffered with bicarbonate and/or HEPES and may include antibiotics and heparin to prevent contamination and clotting.

Micromanipulation procedure: Micromanipulation procedures, including ICSI, are performed outside of the incubator over the objective lens of an inverted microscope **(Table 1)**. Gametes are placed into media drops that are overlaid with light mineral oil, using shallow, sterile, tissue-culture-grade plastic Petri dishes. The microtools used for these procedures are constructed from borosilicate glass capillary tubes, which are essential for holding oocytes and aspirating or injecting spermatozoa.

Micromanipulation systems attached to an inverted microscope, requiring specific equipment and conditions due to the setup's limited working distance include:

- *Precision micromanipulators:* Micromanipulation systems, either hydraulic or motorized, provide high precision in the movement of microinjection and holding pipettes. Hydraulic micromanipulators are preferred for their smooth, backlash-free movement, ensuring fine control during ICSI.
- *Objective lens and working distance:* The inverted microscope's objective lens has a limited working distance, necessitating the use of low-profile micromanipulation tools. This space constraint demands specialized, finely designed pipettes that can operate efficiently within the microscope's field without obstructing visibility or movement.
- *Microenvironment maintenance:* During micromanipulation, maintaining optimal conditions is critical. A heated stage is used to regulate the temperature of the gametes and culture media at physiological levels (37°C), which minimizes temperature-induced stress and ensures the viability of the oocyte and spermatozoa throughout the procedure.
- *High-resolution imaging:* The inverted microscope is typically equipped with advanced imaging systems, such as differential interference contrast (DIC) or Hoffman modulation contrast, which enhance the visibility of cells

TABLE 1: Overview of micromanipulator systems and microinjectors used in intracytoplasmic sperm injection (ICSI).

Type of micromanipulator system	*Control system*	*Scientific points*
Motorized micromanipulator	Motorized	• Utilizes electric motors for precise control • Suitable for complex and automated movements • Can be integrated with digital systems for enhanced precision
Manual micromanipulator	Manual	• Requires manual adjustment for movement • Provides high control but is user-dependent • More suitable for basic procedures with fewer complexities
Automatic micromanipulator	Automated	• Features computer-controlled automation • Ensures high reproducibility and precision • Ideal for high-throughput ICSI procedures
Piezo micromanipulator	Piezoelectric control	• Uses piezoelectric crystals for movement • Offers rapid and precise movements with minimal vibration • Highly effective for delicate procedures like ICSI
Hydraulic microinjector (holding/injecting)	Hydraulic	• Utilizes fluid pressure for holding and injecting cells • Provides smooth, precise control • Requires regular maintenance to prevent fluid leakage
Pneumatic microinjector (holding/injecting)	Pneumatic	• Operates using air pressure for holding and injecting cells • Offers high precision with minimal mechanical interference • Less sensitive to vibrations

and subcellular structures, improving the precision of microinjections and manipulations during ICSI.

- *Use of specialized pipettes:* Micropipettes used in ICSI, including injection and holding pipettes, are designed with specific dimensions to suit the oocyte's structure. The injection pipette's diameter, typically 5–10 µm, allows for smooth sperm insertion, while the holding pipette stabilizes the oocyte without causing mechanical damage.
- *Vibration control:* To enhance precision, micromanipulation systems are often placed on anti-vibration tables, which minimize external mechanical disturbances that could affect the accuracy of the micromanipulation process. Vibrations, even at low frequencies, can lead to errors during sperm injection or oocyte handling.
- *Three-dimensional control:* The micromanipulator system allows for precise three-dimensional movement, controlled via joystick or precision knobs, enabling the operator to manipulate sperm and oocytes accurately. This level of control is essential for minimizing oocyte damage

and increasing the success rates of fertilization in ICSI procedures.

- *Operator skill:* The success of micromanipulation procedures like ICSI is highly dependent on the skill and experience of the operator. Proper handling of the micromanipulation system requires extensive training to ensure accurate sperm injection and minimize potential damage to the oocyte membrane.
- *Micromanipulation environment:* The entire process occurs in an open system, outside the controlled environment of an incubator. Therefore, the microscope stage is heated, and media are supplemented with essential nutrients and stabilizers to mimic in vivo conditions as closely as possible, ensuring the maintenance of cell viability during the procedure.

Intracytoplasmic sperm injection technique: The same media used for oocyte preparation are employed during micromanipulation. However, when procedures extend outside the incubator for longer durations, a HEPES-buffered medium supplemented with penicillin, pyruvate, and human serum albumin (HSA) is recommended. Polyvinylpyrrolidone (PVP) is commonly used for sperm manipulation due to its capacity to reduce sperm motility, making the spermatozoa easier to inject.

The ICSI involves the precise injection of a morphologically normal sperm into an oocyte. To ensure success, the laboratory environment must be free from vibrations to prevent disruptions during the procedure.

Manipulation of the spermatozoon: The ICSI process is conducted using a micromanipulator attached to an inverted microscope. The spermatozoon must be completely immobilized, which is achieved by damaging its tail. This step is crucial and is done by aligning the sperm with the injection needle and intentionally breaking the tail. The sperm is then aspirated and positioned at the tip of the injection needle for subsequent injection **(Figs. 1 to 4)**.

Manipulation of the oocyte: The oocyte is prepared for injection by positioning its polar body at either the 12 o'clock or 6 o'clock position **(Fig. 5)**. The spermatozoon is carefully placed at the tip of the injection needle, and the geometric center of the oocyte is identified by gently indenting the zona pellucida **(Fig. 6)**. The needle is then pushed horizontally through the zona pellucida and vitelline membrane, creating an invagination **(Fig. 7)**. A precise

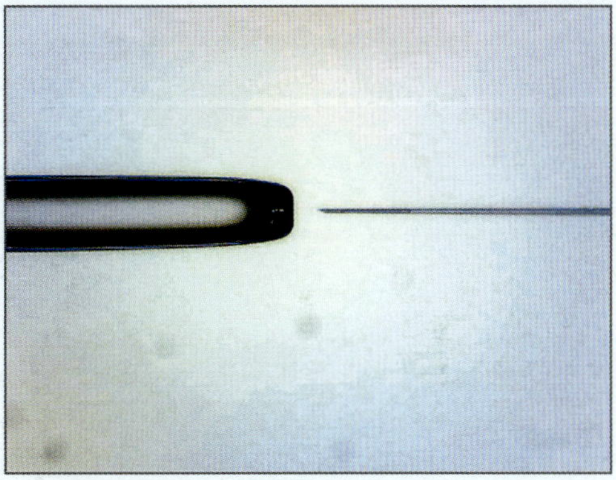

Fig. 1: Precisely aligned holding and injection pipettes.

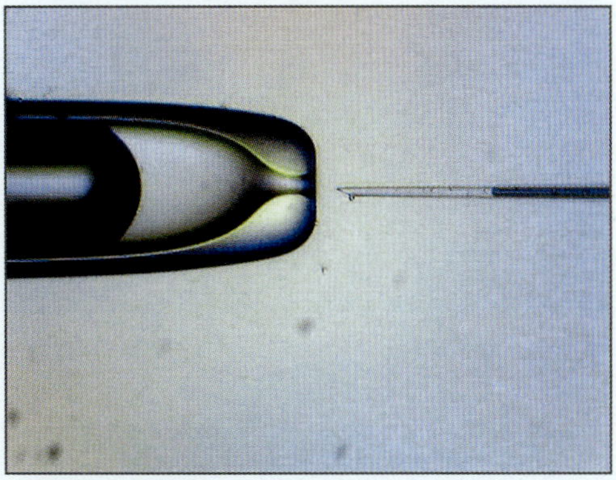

Fig. 2: Pipettes immersed in media drop for washing and pressure calibration.

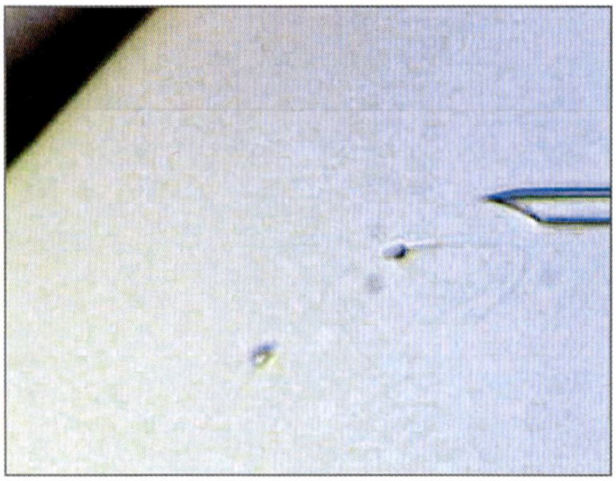

Fig. 3: The sperm tail is slashed to partially immobilize and assess morphology.

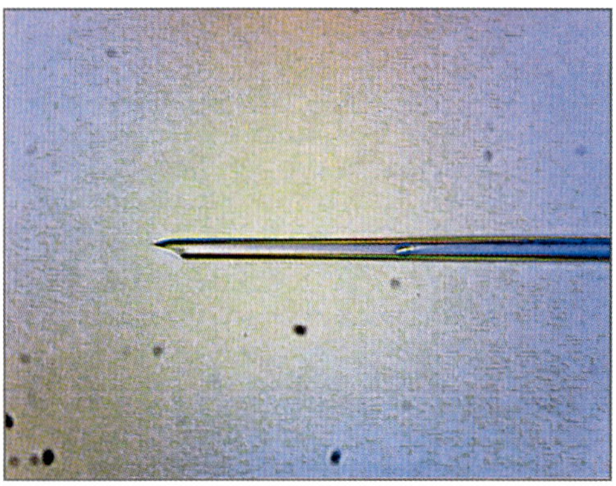

Fig. 4: Carefully aspirate the tapped sperm into the micropipette.

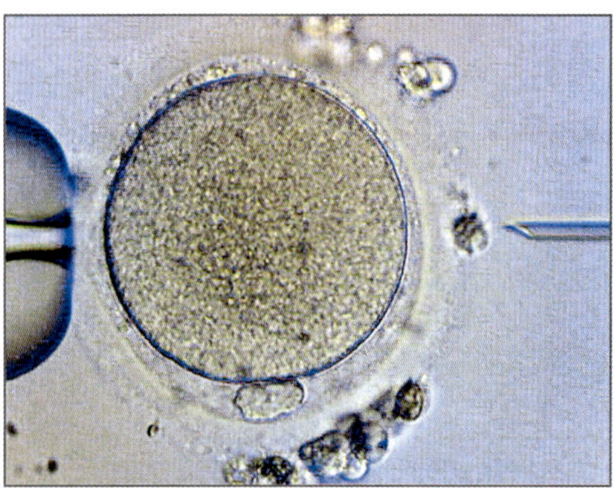

Fig. 5: Position the oocyte so that the polar body is at either the 6 o'clock or 12 o'clock position.

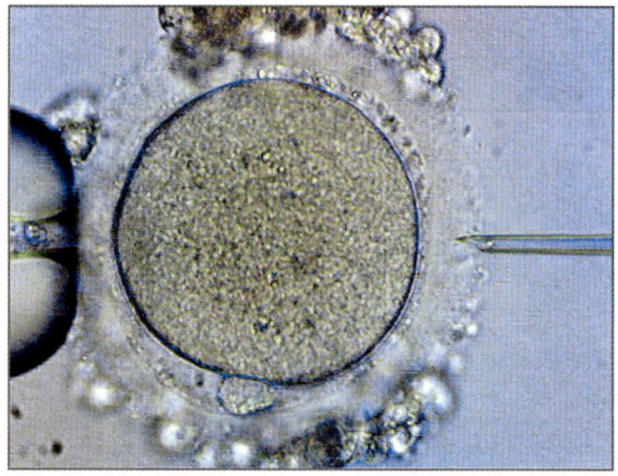

Fig. 6: Secure the oocyte firmly and position the sperm precisely at the tip for injection from the 3 o'clock position.

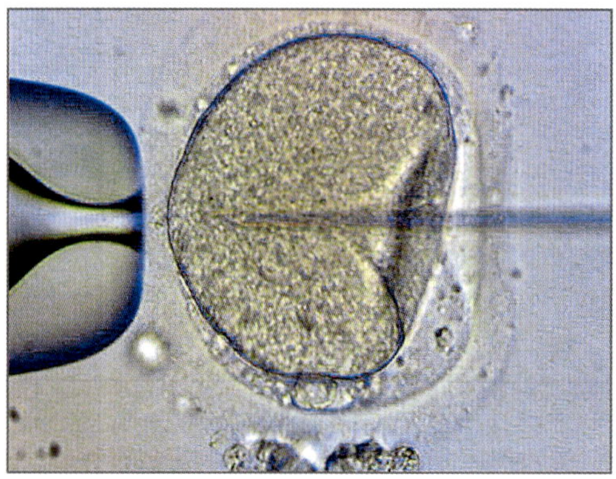

Fig. 7: Inject the oocyte until the pipette reaches the 9 o'clock position, aspirate some cytoplasm until breakage is observed, and then deposit the sperm.

jab from the 3 o'clock position is used to break the membrane, and a small amount of cytoplasmic material is aspirated to ensure the needle is correctly positioned within the cytosol. The spermatozoon is then deposited at the 9 o'clock position **(Fig. 8)**.

Following injection, the oocytes are transferred to preincubated culture medium layered with oil and incubated at 37°C in 5% CO_2 for 18–20 hours. Fertilization is assessed post incubation using an inverted microscope. Normally fertilized oocytes will exhibit two pronuclei and two polar bodies.

The cleavage of these fertilized oocytes is evaluated on the second day following ICSI.[2]

TROUBLESHOOTING

Troubleshooting during ICSI is essential for overcoming challenges that can occur during the delicate sperm injection process. By quickly identifying and resolving issues like pipette blockages, improper sperm immobilization, or difficulty penetrating the oocyte membrane, embryologists can improve the chances of successful fertilization and achieve better clinical outcomes **(Table 2)**.

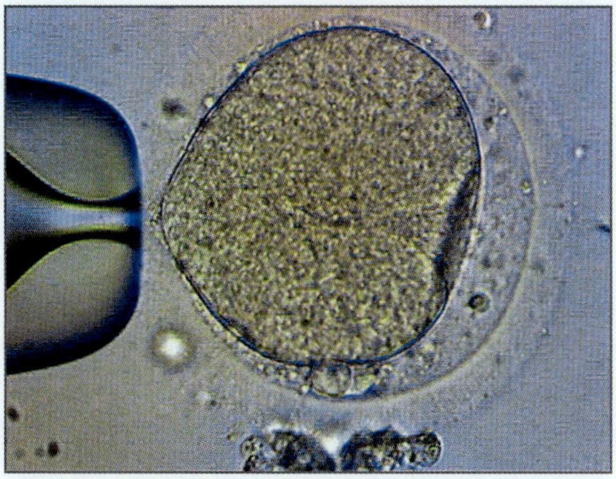

Fig. 8: Withdraw the microinjection pipette and gently release the oocyte.

CONCLUSION

The ICSI procedure, while intricate and demanding, is a critical component of assisted reproductive technology. The success of ICSI not only hinges on the precision of the micromanipulation techniques but also on the delicate handling and preparation of oocytes and spermatozoa. Ensuring optimal environmental conditions and using appropriate media throughout the procedure are vital for enhancing fertilization outcomes and improving embryo quality, ultimately

TABLE 2: Common intracytoplasmic sperm injection (ICSI) issues and troubleshooting steps.

Issue	*Description*	*Troubleshooting steps*
Difficulty immobilizing spermatozoa	Spermatozoa continue to move after tail damage, complicating the injection process	• Ensure complete tail severance with additional force • Use polyvinylpyrrolidone (PVP) to reduce sperm motility • Check the sharpness and alignment of the injection needle
Problems with oocyte handling	Oocytes are difficult to hold or manipulate due to slippage or movement	• Adjust holding pipette suction strength • Reposition the holding pipette for a better grip • Ensure proper medium viscosity to prevent movement
Difficulty penetrating the zona pellucida	Injection needle fails to penetrate the zona pellucida smoothly	• Confirm needle sharpness and inspect for deformities • Adjust the angle of entry to be perpendicular • Apply consistent pressure during insertion
Improper positioning of the oocyte's polar body	Polar body is not correctly aligned, risking oocyte damage	• Rotate the oocyte using the micromanipulator • Adjust microscope optics and lighting for better visualization • Reposition the holding pipette

Contd...

Contd...

Issue	***Description***	***Troubleshooting steps***
Inconsistent needle insertion	Injection needle does not enter the cytoplasm smoothly, leading to failed injection	• Ensure micromanipulator calibration and smooth operation • Practice gentle, controlled needle movements • Reattempt insertion with proper alignment if resistance is felt
Difficulty aspirating cytoplasmic material	There is trouble confirming needle placement in the cytoplasm	• Check suction settings on the micromanipulator • Use a new, clean needle to avoid blockages • Adjust needle depth to ensure it is in the cytoplasmic region
Oocyte degeneration post-ICSI	Oocytes degenerate after the ICSI procedure, leading to failed fertilization	• Review the procedure for potential sources of trauma • Handle oocytes quickly and return them to optimal conditions • Ensure media quality and avoid contamination
Vibration interference during ICSI	Vibrations in the laboratory affect micromanipulation stability	• Use vibration isolation platforms • Regularly maintain the micromanipulator • Minimize movement around the workstation during the procedure

contributing to higher pregnancy rates. As such, continuous advancements in the protocols and techniques used in ICSI are essential for optimizing the success of this procedure in clinical practice.

REFERENCES

1. Palermo G, et al. The first successful ICSI embryo and pregnancy. Reprod Med J. 1992.
2. Smith A, et al. Advancements in ICSI techniques. J Assist Reprod Genet. 2022.
3. Jones B, et al. Technical aspects of ICSI in assisted reproduction. Reprod Biol Endocrinol. 2021.
4. Brown C, et al. Handling and preparation of oocytes for ICSI. Fertil Steril. 2020.

12 CHAPTER

Fertilization Assessment and Embryo Grading

INTRODUCTION

Fertilization assessment globally follows standardized protocols, typically involving the identification of two pronuclei and polar bodies within 16–18 hours post insemination, ensuring normal fertilization. Embryo grading systems, such as those from the ESHRE (European Society of Human Reproduction and Embryology), ASRM (American Society for Reproductive Medicine), and Istanbul Consensus, emphasize parameters like cell count, symmetry, fragmentation, and blastocyst development to uniformly assess embryo quality for transfer, cryopreservation, or further culture. These grading systems aim to optimize embryo selection for successful implantation and pregnancy outcomes worldwide **(Table 1)**.

FERTILIZATION ASSESSMENT AND PRONUCLEAR SCORING

Optimal fertilization of oocytes is critical for successful embryo development. An ideally fertilized oocyte should be spherical, contain two polar bodies, and have two centrally located, juxtaposed pronuclei of equal size with distinct membranes.[1] The pronuclei should have equal numbers and sizes of nucleolar precursor bodies (NPBs), ideally aligned equatorially at the region where the membranes meet.

Fertilization check: At the fertilization check, both the size and location of the pronuclei should be evaluated. Features such as widely separated pronuclei, pronuclei of significantly different sizes, and the presence of micronuclei are considered severely atypical. If smooth endoplasmic reticulum (sER) disks are observed in normally fertilized oocytes (especially after conventional In vitro fertilization (IVF) rather than ICSI), these oocytes should not be used for transfer.

Second day-1 assessment: A second assessment on day 1 may be conducted for quality control or prognostic reasons, focusing either on syngamy or early cleavage.[1]

Pronuclear scoring: Pronuclear scoring provides additional information to the fertilization check **(Figs. 1A to D)**. It categorizes pronuclei as symmetrical, nonsymmetrical, or abnormal. Abnormal pronuclei include those with no NPBs (ghost pronuclei) and those with a single NPB (bull's eye pronuclei), which are associated with poor outcomes.[2]

CLEAVAGE-STAGE EMBRYOS

Assessment of cell number: Embryos should be at specific developmental stages at set times post insemination: 4 cells on day 2 and 8 cells on day 3. Deviation from these rates is linked to reduced implantation potential.[1]

Fragmentation: Fragments, defined as extracellular membrane-bound cytoplasmic structures, are categorized by severity: Mild (<10%), moderate (10–25%), and severe (>25%). Fragment size also varies by the embryo's stage: <45 μm in diameter on day 2

TABLE 1: Fertilization assessment and embryo grading as per various consensus worldwide.

Grading system	*Year*	*Criteria*	*Grades*	*Description*
Zygote scoring (Z-Score)	1999	Pronuclei alignment, nucleolar precursor bodies (NPBs)	Z1 to Z4	• *Z1:* Perfect alignment of pronuclei and NPBs • *Z2:* Slight deviation in alignment • *Z3:* Pronuclei and NPBs are not aligned • *Z4*: Pronuclei and NPBs are highly misaligned
Day-3 cleavage-stage grading	1988	Cell number, symmetry, fragmentation	1–4	• *Grade 1:* 6–8 cells, no fragmentation, symmetric • *Grade 2:* 6–8 cells, <10% fragmentation, slightly asymmetric • *Grade 3:* 6–8 cells, 10–25% fragmentation • *Grade 4:* <6 cells, >25% fragmentation, highly asymmetric
Day-5 blastocyst grading	1999	Expansion, inner cell (ICM) mass, trophectoderm (TE)	1–6 (expansion), A to C (ICM and TE)	• *Expansion (1–6):* 1 = Early blastocyst, 6 = Hatching blastocyst • *ICM (A to C):* A = Tightly packed, B = Loosely packed, C = Few cells • *TE (A to C):* A = Many cells, B = Few cells, C = Very few cells
SART (Society for Assisted Reproductive Technology) grading	2000	Cell number, fragmentation, symmetry	Excellent, good, fair, poor	• *Excellent:* 6–8 cells, <10% fragmentation, symmetric • *Good:* 6–8 cells, 10–20% fragmentation, slightly asymmetric • *Fair:* 5–8 cells, 20–50% fragmentation, moderately asymmetric • *Poor:* <5 cells, >50% fragmentation, highly asymmetric
ASRM (American Society for Reproductive Medicine) Grading	2000	Cell number, fragmentation, symmetry, multinucleation	1–4	• *Grade 1:* 6–8 cells, <10% fragmentation, symmetric, no multinucleation • *Grade 2:* 6–8 cells, 10–25% fragmentation, slightly asymmetric, no multinucleation • *Grade 3:* 5–8 cells, 25–50% fragmentation, moderately asymmetric, possible multinucleation • *Grade 4:* <5 cells, >50% fragmentation, highly asymmetric, multinucleation present
Gardner's blastocyst grading	2000	Expansion, ICM, TE	1–6 (expansion), A to C (ICM and TE)	• *Expansion (1–6):* 1 = Early blastocyst, 6 = Fully expanded • *ICM (A to C):* A = Many cells, B = Several cells, C = Few cells • *TE (A to C):* A = Many cells forming a cohesive epithelium, B = Few cells forming a loose epithelium, C = Very few cells

Contd...

Contd...

Grading system	***Year***	***Criteria***	***Grades***	***Description***
Alpha Scientists and ESHRE (European Society of Human Reproduction and Embryology)	2011	Comprehensive morphology evaluation	Different categories	This evaluates cumulus–corona complex, cytoplasm, polar body, and overall morphology to categorize oocytes into different grades

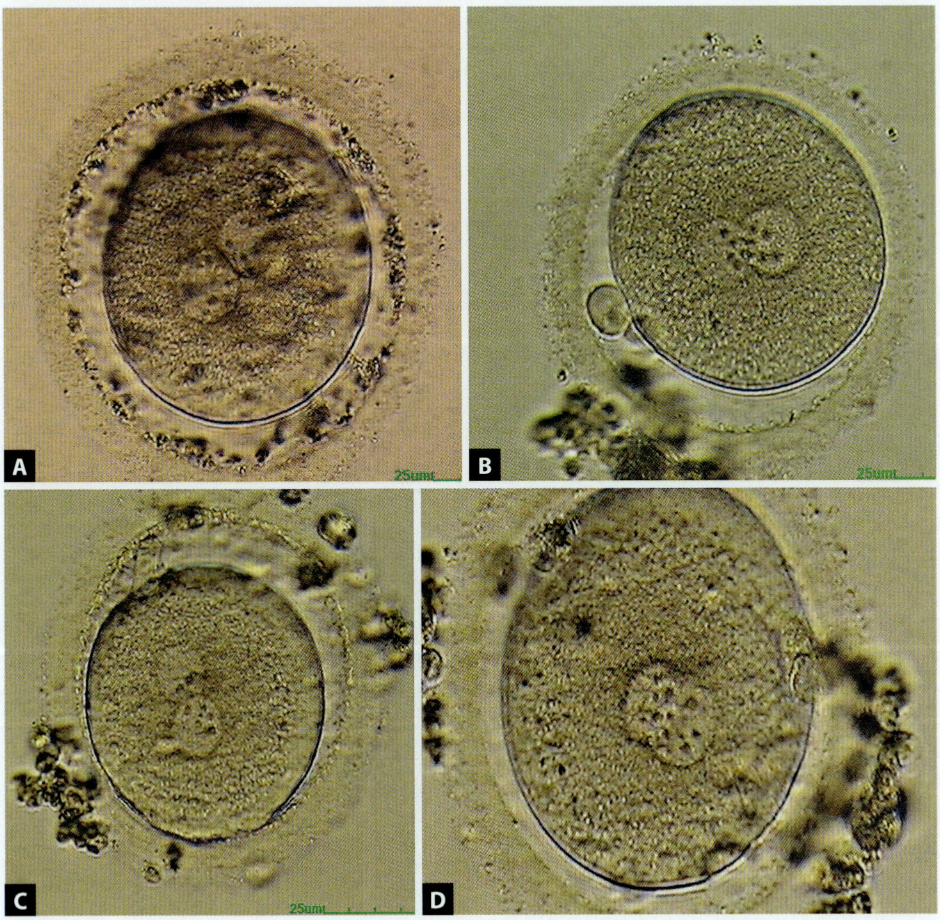

Figs. 1A to D: Fertilization assessment: Confirmation of normal fertilization with presence of 2 pronuclei.

and <40 μm on day 3. The impact of fragment localization is not clearly defined due to its dynamic nature within the embryo.

Multinucleation: Multinucleation, the presence of more than one nucleus in a blastomere, is linked to decreased implantation potential and increased chromosomal abnormalities. Multinucleated embryos have a higher risk of spontaneous abortion. Assessment is recommended on day 2

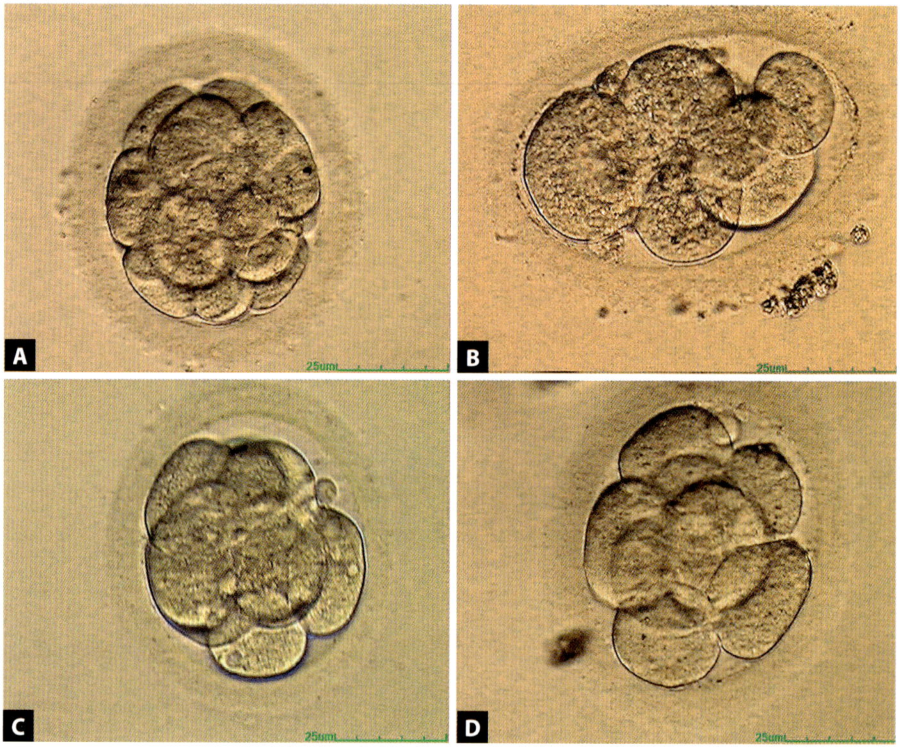

Figs. 2A to D: Day-3 cleavage-stage embryo assessment revealing embryos at the 6–8 cell stage.

(44 ± 1 h post insemination). Recording the incidence of multinucleation in each embryo is essential for accurate evaluation.[1]

Cell size and other morphological features: For embryos at the 2-, 4-, and 8-cell stages, blastomeres should be evenly sized. Other stages may show size differences due to incomplete cleavage phases. Cytoplasmic granularity, membrane appearance, and vacuoles are also assessed, though their impact on implantation potential requires further research.

Cleavage-stage embryo scoring system: An optimal day-2 embryo (44 ± 1 h post insemination) should have four equally sized mononucleated blastomeres in a three-dimensional tetrahedral arrangement, with <10% fragmentation. For day-3 embryos (68 ± 1 h post insemination), an optimal embryo should have eight equally sized mononucleated blastomeres with <10% fragmentation **(Figs. 2A to D)**.[1] The scoring system for cleavage-stage embryos includes cell number, grade, and reason for the grade.

DAY-4 AND DAY-5 ASSESSMENTS

Day-4 assessment (morula stage): A day-4 embryo should be compacted or compacting, entering the fourth round of cleavage. Compaction should involve nearly all the embryo volume **(Figs. 3A and B)**. The consensus scoring system for day-4 embryos includes grades for good, fair, and poor embryos based on the extent of compaction.[3]

Day-5 assessment (blastocyst stage): At this stage (116 ± 2 h post insemination),

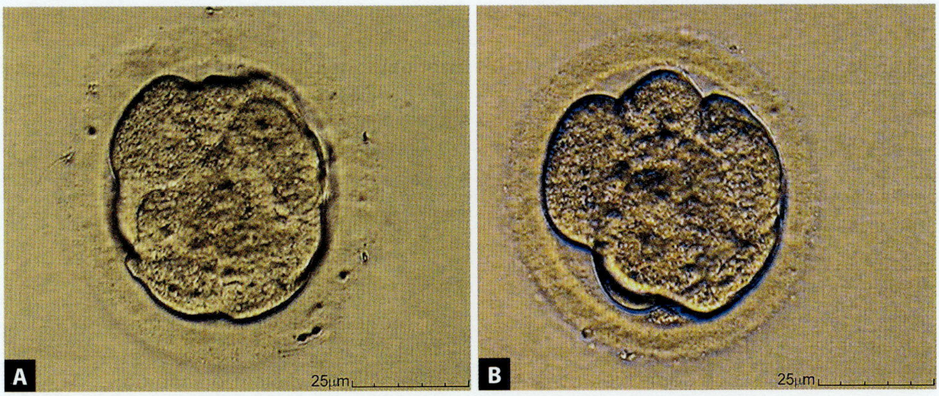

Figs. 3A and B: Day-4 assessment: Morula stage embryos.

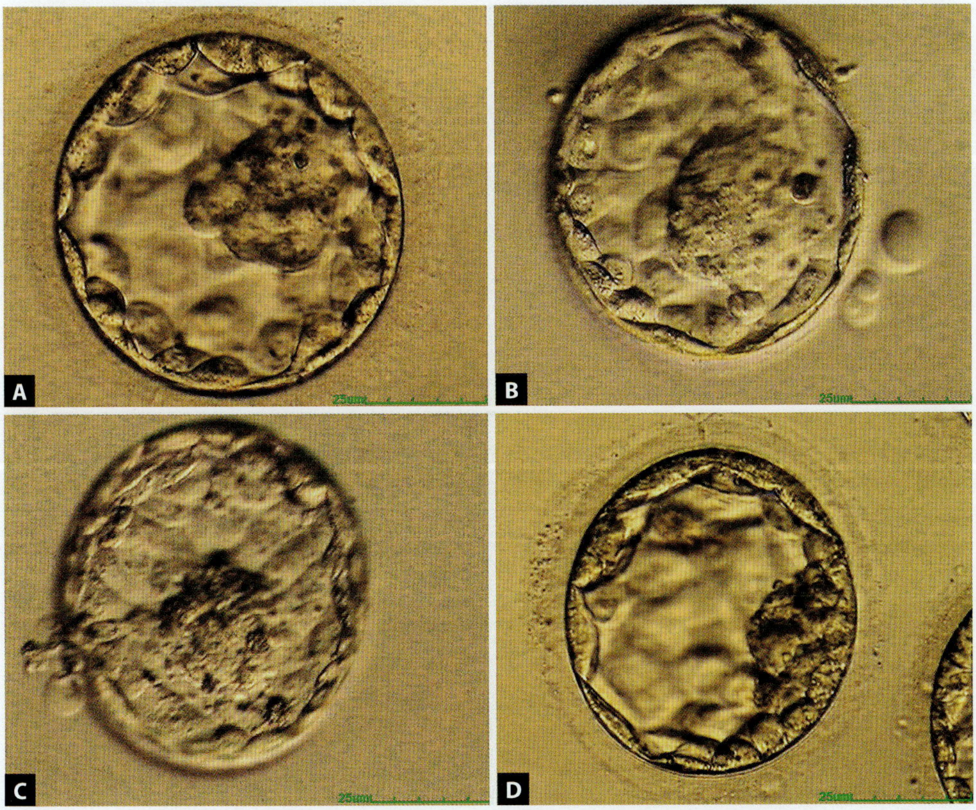

Figs. 4A to D: Day-5 assessment: Expanded blastocyst observed.

an optimal blastocyst should be fully expanded to hatched, with a prominent, easily discernible inner cell mass (ICM) and a cohesive trophectoderm (TE).[4] The ICM and TE are crucial for implantation and fetal development **(Figs. 4A to D)**. Variants like cytoplasmic strings or structures in the perivitelline space have unknown significance and require further investigation.

Definition of a nonviable embryo: A nonviable embryo is defined as one where development has arrested for at least 24 hours, or where all cells have degenerated or lysed.[1]

These consensus points aim to standardize the assessment of oocyte and embryo morphology worldwide, fostering a common language among embryologists.

CONCLUSION

Paying close attention to how we assess fertilization and grade embryos is crucial for the success of assisted reproductive technology (ART) procedures. By following consistent guidelines for evaluating each stage—from pronuclei to blastocysts—embryologists can better predict, which embryos are most likely to result in a successful pregnancy. This approach requires not only precision but also a willingness to adapt to new research and techniques. By doing so, ART laboratories can improve their success rates, offering better outcomes and hope for patients looking to start or grow their families.

REFERENCES

1. Alpha Scientists in Reproductive Medicine and ESHRE Special Interest Group of Embryology. The Istanbul consensus workshop on embryo assessment: Expert meeting proceedings. Hum Reprod. 2011; 26(6):1270-8.
2. Scott L. Pronuclear scoring as a predictor of embryo development. Reprod Biomed Online. 2003;6(2):201-14.
3. Tao J, et al. Compaction patterns in day 4 embryos and their relationship with implantation potential. Fertil Steril. 2002; 78(5):1096-100.
4. Gardner DK, Schoolcraft WB. Culture and transfer of human blastocysts. Curr Opin Obstet Gynecol. 1999;11(3):307-11.

CHAPTER 13

Selection of Embryos for Transfer

INTRODUCTION

Embryo selection for transfer is a critical step in assisted reproductive technology (ART), aimed at maximizing the chances of implantation and successful pregnancy. The process involves assessing embryos based on developmental stages, morphological quality, and, in some cases, genetic integrity. Advances such as preimplantation genetic diagnosis (PGD) have revealed the limitations of relying solely on morphology, highlighting the importance of combining visual assessment with genetic screening. The timing of embryo transfer, whether at the cleavage stage (Day 2 or 3) or the blastocyst stage (Day 5), plays a crucial role, with each offering unique advantages and considerations. Meticulous preparation, careful handling, and the use of advanced tools ensure a smooth, atraumatic transfer, which is vital for optimal outcomes.

CRITERIA FOR EMBRYO SELECTION

Traditionally, embryo transfer is performed on day 2, approximately 48 hours postfertilization. However, delaying transfer until day 3, about 69–72 hours postfertilization, has not shown detrimental effects on pregnancy rates and may aid in selecting embryos with better prognosis.[1] Day 5 blastocyst transfer offers its own advantages and disadvantages, requiring stringent and homogeneous culture conditions. A significant concern is the fate of day 3 embryos that fail to form grade one blastocysts by day 5, which might otherwise result in successful pregnancies.

TIMING AND STAGES OF EMBRYO TRANSFER

When selecting embryos for transfer, the timing of observation and judgment is crucial, as it captures a single moment in a rapidly developing process **(Table 1)**. Generally, embryos at later stages and higher grades are preferred. Fragmentation patterns and the appearance of the zona pellucida are also important considerations. Embryos demonstrating grade-one to grade-two qualities throughout development are prioritized for transfer, while grade-three and four embryos are considered only if higher grade embryos are unavailable.[1]

TABLE 1: Embryo developmental stages and time of transfer.

Timing postinsemination	*Day*	*Embryo stage*
48–50 hours	Day 2	2–4 cell stage
69–72 hours	Day 3	8–10 cell stage
116–120 hours	Day 5	Expanded blastocyst stage

Source: Alpha Scientists in Reproductive Medicine and ESHRE Special Interest Group of Embryology. The Istanbul consensus workshop on embryo assessment: expert meeting proceedings. Hum Reprod. 2011;26(6):1270-8.

GENETIC SCREENING AND EMBRYO SELECTION

The application of preimplantation genetic diagnosis (PGD) utilizing fluorescence in situ hybridization (FISH) on biopsied blastomeres has illuminated discrepancies between the morphological assessment and genetic integrity of embryos. Research by Munné (2002) has demonstrated that embryos deemed morphologically optimal may still harbor underlying genetic abnormalities, while those exhibiting fragmentation can retain normal implantation potential. This underscores the limitations of relying solely on visual criteria for embryo selection. Consequently, embryos that remain following the transfer are often cryopreserved, preserving their potential for future use in subsequent assisted reproductive technology (ART) cycles.[2]

EMBRYO TRANSFER PROCEDURE

Typically, a maximum of two embryos are transferred, though in exceptional cases, three may be transferred.

Preparation and Procedure

The embryo-loaded catheter and syringe are handed to the clinician for transfer. Postprocedure, the catheter is flushed under a microscope to ensure no embryo remains trapped in mucus or blood. If any embryo is retained, it should be reloaded into a fresh clean catheter, and the transfer procedure should be repeated.[1]

In case of complications during transfer, causing delays, embryos should be returned to the culture environment and transferred later. Performing a traumatic transfer must be avoided as it can induce uterine contractions and prostaglandin release, potentially washing off embryos or causing infections if bleeding occurs.

Patient Preparation

A trial transfer in the previous cycle is recommended to anticipate and address potential difficulties. Patients are instructed not to urinate for an hour before the transfer and to avoid using vaginal progesterone pessaries. During the procedure, the patient is positioned in the lithotomy position, and a transabdominal ultrasound is performed to ensure a full bladder and clear visualization of the endometrium. The cervix is then cleaned of excess discharge or mucus with a swab moistened in culture medium, and the speculum is adjusted for optimal cervical canal access.

Catheter Insertion

Embryos are loaded into the catheter with culture medium and air bubbles for visualization **(Table 2)**. The catheter is carefully introduced into the cervical canal, avoiding contact with the vaginal wall. Once the catheter tip is visualized near the internal os, it is gently advanced 1–1.5 cm from the fundus, and the embryos are gently expelled into the uterine cavity, visible via ultrasound as tiny bubbles.[3]

Importance of Atraumatic Transfer

Ensuring the embryo transfer is as atraumatic as possible is crucial for successful pregnancy outcomes. Careful handling and minimal cervical manipulation are key to preventing uterine contractions and potential embryo loss.[1]

CONCLUSION

Embryo transfer is a delicate procedure that requires careful timing and consideration of embryo quality. Advances in genetic screening have highlighted the complexity of embryo selection, emphasizing the need for both morphological and genetic

TABLE 2: Embryo transfer catheters: A detailed comparison of types, characteristics, and usage difficulty.

Catheter	*Type*	*Soft/hard*	*Description*	*Difficulty*
SureView	Single lumen	Soft	A popular soft catheter with an echogenic tip for improved visibility during transfer	Low
EchoTip	Single lumen	Soft	Soft catheter with an echogenic tip, designed for gentle placement and reduced trauma	Low
Embryo transfer catheter	Single lumen	Hard	A more rigid catheter designed for easier passage in cases of difficult cervical anatomy	Medium
Embryo transfer catheter	Single lumen	Soft	A soft catheter known for its flexibility and gentle handling of embryos during transfer	Low
Double-lumen IVF (in vitro fertilization)	Double lumen	Soft	A double-lumen catheter that allows for flushing if necessary, with a soft design for delicate transfers	Medium
Memory function	Single lumen	Soft	A soft catheter designed with a memory function to retain its shape during transfer	Low
Nano-Kat	Single lumen	Hard	A thin, rigid catheter designed for cases requiring precise navigation through difficult anatomy	High
Classic	Single lumen	Soft	Known for its reliability and ease of use, with a gentle design to minimize trauma	Low
EchoTip	Single lumen	Hard	A rigid catheter designed for use with ultrasound guidance, offering precise control in challenging transfers	Medium
Double-lumen ETR	Double lumen	Soft	Designed for both embryo transfer and fluid aspiration, this soft catheter offers versatility in ART procedures	Medium

(ART: assisted reproductive technology; ETR: catheter)

assessments. The procedure's success hinges on meticulous preparation and execution, ensuring the best possible outcomes for patients.

REFERENCES

1. Alpha Scientists in Reproductive Medicine and ESHRE Special Interest Group of Embryology. The Istanbul consensus workshop on embryo assessment: expert meeting proceedings. Hum Reprod. 2011; 26(6): 1270-8.
2. Munné S. Preimplantation genetic diagnosis of structural, numerical, and polyploid chromosomal abnormalities. Reprod Biomed Online. 2002;6(2):227-35.
3. Gardner DK, Schoolcraft WB. Culture and transfer of human blastocysts. Curr Opin Obstet Gynecol. 1999;11(3):307-11.

CHAPTER 14

Blastocyst Culture and Transfer

INTRODUCTION

Blastocyst culture and transfer have significantly enhanced the take-home baby rates in assisted reproductive technology (ART) worldwide. In a naturally fertile woman, oocytes are fertilized, and the resulting embryo undergoes cleavage to reach the compacted or cavitated stages (day 4 to 5) within the fallopian tube. The embryo then descends into the uterus for further development, including hatching from the zona pellucida (ZP) and implantation, typically occurring between days 5 and 7.[1]

Besides the synchrony of the blastocyst stage with the uterine environment, there are numerous other advantages to performing blastocyst transfers.

CULTURE CONDITIONS FOR BLASTOCYST

The metabolic requirements of human embryos vary significantly from one stage to another. To meet these changing needs, commercially available sequential media are used. For optimal blastocyst culture, the media should contain high concentrations of glucose, selected nonessential and essential amino acids, macromolecules, increased levels of magnesium, and lactate. The medium should be free of phosphate, ethylenediaminetetraacetic acid (EDTA), and taurine. This combination supports robust blastocyst development.[2]

ADVANTAGES OF BLASTOCYST CULTURE

Blastocyst culture offers multiple benefits, including:

- *Enhanced viability:* By overcoming the in vitro development block between day 2 and 3, blastocyst culture produces the most viable embryos for transfer.[3]
- *Selection of hardy embryos:* Genetically defective embryos typically cease development, allowing only the hardiest embryos to survive longer in vitro, resulting in a more selective population for replacement.[4]
- *Physiological synchrony:* Transferring blastocyst-stage embryos into the uterus provides a more physiological environment compared to transferring earlier cleavage-stage embryos.[5]
- *Genetic integrity:* Blastocyst culture reduces the risk of inheriting an abnormal paternal genome, particularly following intracytoplasmic sperm injection (ICSI).[6]
- *Noninvasive assessment:* Indirect, non-invasive microscopic assessment of blastocysts for high total cell numbers can be used to select the most viable embryos before transfer.[7]
- *Improved implantation:* Complete removal of the ZP at the blastocyst stage, followed by the transfer of zona-free blastocysts, may promote better and direct anchorage of the trophectoderm

to the endometrial epithelium, thereby improving implantation rates.[8]

- *Post-thaw evaluation:* When freezing pronuclear and cleavage stage embryos, blastocyst culture allows for a period of evaluation post-thaw, facilitating embryo recovery and subsequent replacement.[9]
- *Embryo repair:* The culture period aids in the repair process of embryos after micromanipulation procedures such as ICSI, embryo biopsy, and assisted hatching.[10]
- *Reduced interval to implantation:* Transferring blastocysts into the uterus reduces the time interval between embryo growth and implantation.[11]
- *Stem cell source:* Blastocyst culture provides a source of inner cell mass (ICM) cells for developing human embryonic stem cells.[12]

TECHNIQUES FOR BLASTOCYST TRANSFER

Considerations for Single Blastocyst Transfer

Single blastocyst transfer (SBT) is increasingly recommended to reduce the risk of multiple pregnancies, which can carry higher risks for both the mother and the babies. SBT is particularly encouraged when a high-quality blastocyst is available, as it can achieve similar pregnancy rates to the transfer of multiple embryos while minimizing the associated risks.[4]

Advances in Blastocyst Transfer Techniques

Recent advances have enhanced the precision and success rates of blastocyst transfers. These include the use of time-lapse imaging to continuously monitor embryo development, allowing for the selection of the most viable blastocyst, and the improvement of catheter design for more efficient and less traumatic transfers.[11] Additionally, the development of blastocyst vitrification techniques has enabled high survival rates of cryopreserved blastocysts, providing more flexible options for transfer timing.[9]

CONCLUSION

Blastocyst culture and transfer have revolutionized assisted reproductive technology by aligning the embryo's developmental stage with the uterine environment, enhancing implantation potential and pregnancy rates. By utilizing advanced culture systems and techniques, including single blastocyst transfer and vitrification, the procedure minimizes risks such as multiple pregnancies while maximizing efficiency. These advancements not only improve clinical outcomes but also provide flexibility in treatment, ensuring better prospects for patients undergoing fertility treatments.

REFERENCES

1. Gardner DK, Lane M, Stevens J, Schoolcraft WB. Blastocyst score affects implantation and pregnancy outcome: towards a single blastocyst transfer. Fertil Steril. 1998;69(1): 84-92.
2. Biggers JD, Racowsky C, Edwards RG. Evolution of the sequential media concept for culturing preimplantation embryos. Reprod Biomed Online. 2002;4(2):133-42.
3. Gardner DK, Lane M. Development of viable mammalian embryos in vitro: evolution of sequential media. Adv Exp Med Biol. 2004;543:45-61.
4. Balaban B, Urman B, Alatas C, Aksoy S, Mercan R, Isiklar A, et al. Blastocyst embryo transfer increases implantation and pregnancy rates in patients undergoing intracytoplasmic sperm injection. J Assist Reprod Genet. 2008;18(8):482-6.

5. Gardner DK, Lane M. Culture and selection of viable blastocysts: a feasible proposition for human IVF? Hum Reprod Update. 1997;3(4):367-82.
6. Mantikou E, Wong KM, Repping S, Mastenbroek S. Molecular origin of mitotic aneuploidies in preimplantation embryos. Biochim Biophys Acta. 2012; 1822(12): 1921-30.
7. Guerif F, Le Gouge A, Giraudeau B, Poindron J, Bidault R, Gasnier O, et al. Limited value of morphological assessment at day 5. Hum Reprod. 2007;22(2):567-74.
8. Van Soom A, Mateusen B, Leroy J, De Kruif A. Assessment of mammalian embryo quality: what can we learn from embryo morphology? Reprod Biomed Online. 2003; 7(6):664-70.
9. Cobo A, Bellver J, Domingo J, Perez S, Crespo J, Pellicer A, et al. New vitrification protocol for day 3 embryos: Improvement in survival and implantation rates. Fertil Steril. 2012;95(8):275-80.
10. Desai N, Goldberg JM, Austin C, Falcone T, Cohen J. The effect of various micromanipulation procedures and cryopreservation on the implantation potential of a human blastocyst. Reprod Biomed Online. 2010; 21(6):751-62.
11. Rienzi L, Ubaldi F, Iacobelli M, Ferrero S, Minasi MG, Martinez F, et al. Day 3 embryo transfer with combined evaluation at the pronuclear and cleavage stages compares favourably with day 5 blastocyst transfer. Hum Reprod. 2002;17(7):1852-5.
12. Thomson JA, Itskovitz-Eldor J, Shapiro SS, Waknitz MA, Swiergiel JJ, Marshall VS, et al. Embryonic stem cell lines derived from human blastocysts. Science. 1998; 282(5391): 1145-7.

CHAPTER

15

Assisted Hatching

INTRODUCTION

Assisted hatching (AH) is an advanced laboratory technique in assisted reproductive technology (ART) designed to improve the implantation potential of embryos. By creating a precise opening in the zona pellucida—the protective glycoprotein shell surrounding the embryo—assisted hatching facilitates the embryo's hatching process, which is essential for successful uterine implantation. This technique is particularly beneficial for patients with advanced maternal age, repeated repeated in vitro fertilization (IVF) failures, poor embryo quality, or embryos with a thick or hardened zona pellucida. Additionally, it supports implantation in frozen-thawed embryos where the zona pellucida may become less flexible due to cryopreservation. By employing techniques such as mechanical, chemical, laser-assisted, or piezo hatching, AH enhances the likelihood of achieving a successful pregnancy in specific patient populations.

INDICATIONS AND TECHNIQUES

When and Why to Perform Assisted Hatching?

Assisted hatching is a laboratory technique used in assisted ART to enhance the implantation potential of embryos. This procedure involves creating an opening in the zona pellucida (ZP), the glycoprotein shell surrounding the oocyte and early embryo, to facilitate the hatching process necessary for successful implantation.

Indications for AH:

- *Advanced maternal age:* Women over the age of 38 years often produce embryos with a thicker or harder ZP, which can hinder hatching and implantation.[1] AH can help overcome this barrier, increasing the likelihood of successful implantation.
- *Repeated in vitro fertilization (IVF) failures:* For patients who have experienced multiple unsuccessful IVF cycles, AH may be recommended to improve implantation rates. This technique addresses issues related to embryo attachment and penetration of the uterine lining.[2]
- *Poor embryo quality:* Embryos with poor morphological quality, such as those with fragmentation or slow development, may benefit from AH. This technique can assist these embryos in implanting more effectively.[3]
- *Thick ZP:* In some cases, embryos naturally develop a thicker ZP. AH can facilitate the natural hatching process, enhancing the likelihood of successful implantation.[2]
- *Frozen-thawed embryos:* Embryos that have been cryopreserved and then thawed may have a hardened ZP due to the freezing process. AH can assist these embryos in breaking through this shell.[4]

TABLE 1: Types of assisted hatching methods with their advantages and disadvantages.

Type of assisted hatching	*Method*	*Description*	*Advantages*	*Disadvantages*
Mechanical hatching	Zona drilling or partial zona dissection	A microneedle is used to mechanically cut or pierce the zona pellucida	Precise control over the opening size	Requires skilled embryologist
Chemical hatching	Acid Tyrode's solution	A small hole is created in the zona pellucida using a chemical solution that dissolves the zona	Effective and commonly used	Potential damage to embryo cells
Laser-assisted hatching	Laser pulses	A laser beam is used to create a small opening in the zona pellucida	Highly precise, reduced handling of embryo	Requires specialized equipment
Enzymatic hatching	Pronase or other enzymes	Enzymes are used to thin or create an opening in the zona pellucida	Less mechanical stress on the embryo	Risk of excessive zona thinning
Mechanical thinning	Micromanipulation	The zona pellucida is thinned using micromanipulation tools without fully breaching it	Controlled thinning, reduces zona rigidity	May not fully assist hatching in all cases

Techniques of Assisted Hatching

Various techniques are used to perform AH, each with its advantages and limitations **(Table 1)**. The primary goal of all methods is to create a precise opening in the ZP without damaging the embryo.

- *Mechanical hatching:* This technique uses a fine needle or micropipette to create a small hole in the ZP. While effective, it requires high precision to avoid damaging the embryo.[5]
- *Chemical hatching:* Acid Tyrode's solution is used to dissolve a small part of the ZP. This method is relatively easy to perform, but it requires careful control to prevent overexposure, which could harm the embryo.[4]
- *Laser-assisted hatching:* This highly precise and controlled method uses a laser beam to thin or perforate the ZP. It is widely used due to its accuracy and reduced risk of mechanical damage.[6]
- *Piezo technology*: This method employs piezoelectric pulses to create an opening in the ZP. While less common, it offers precision and control similar to laser-assisted hatching.[3]

SUCCESS RATES

The effectiveness of AH varies based on the technique used, the patient's specific circumstances, and the overall quality of the embryos. Several studies have reported increased implantation and pregnancy rates with the use of AH in appropriate candidates.

- *Advanced maternal age:* Studies have shown that AH can significantly improve implantation and pregnancy rates in older women. Schoolcraft et al. demonstrated improved outcomes in this patient group.[1]
- *Repeated IVF failures:* Patients with previous failed IVF attempts have also shown improved success rates with AH. Balaban et al. reported higher

implantation and pregnancy rates in these patients when AH was performed.[2]

- *General IVF population:* While not all studies agree on the universal benefits, a meta-analysis by Sallam et al. indicated that AH could increase the chances of implantation and pregnancy, particularly in specific subgroups such as older women or those with repeated IVF failures.[7]

Overall, AH is a valuable technique in ART, offering increased implantation potential for specific patient groups and embryo conditions. Its application should be tailored to individual patient needs and performed with precision to ensure the best outcomes.

TECHNICAL PROCEDURES

Zona Drilling with Acid Tyrode's Solution

Zona drilling with acid Tyrode's solution is a chemical method of AH. The solution, commercially available with a pH of 2.3–2.5, is used to create a small hole in the ZP. The procedure involves the following steps:

1. *Preparation:* Prepare a microinjection dish containing 50 μL droplets of HEPES/bicarbonate-buffered culture medium, one for equilibrating the holding pipette and one for each embryo. The dish should also contain a large droplet (100–200 μL) of acid Tyrode's solution, overlaid with light paraffin oil, and incubated at 37°C.
2. *Setup:* Mount a holding pipette to one side of the micromanipulation system and a drilling pipette to the other. Prime the holding pipette with medium and backfill the drilling pipette with acid Tyrode's solution using negative pressure.
3. *Embryo placement:* Place the embryos into the microinjection dish, one per droplet of culture medium.
4. *Orientation and drilling:* Using the holding pipette, orient the embryo so that the point of contact between the drilling pipette and the ZP is between adjacent blastomeres. Advance the drilling pipette against the ZP and release acid Tyrode's solution until a breach is formed.
5. *Completion:* Once the ZP ruptures, withdraw the drilling pipette and cease the flow of acid Tyrode's solution. Immediately remove the embryo and wash it through bicarbonate-buffered culture medium.

Zona Dissection with Micropipettes

Zona dissection, or zona tearing, uses micropipettes to pierce the ZP. The procedure involves the following steps:

1. *Preparation:* Prepare a microinjection dish with 50 μL droplets of HEPES/bicarbonate-buffered culture medium, overlaid with light paraffin oil, and incubated at 37°C.
2. *Setup:* Mount a holding pipette and an injection pipette on the micromanipulation system. Prime the holding pipette with medium.
3. *Embryo placement:* Place the embryos into the microinjection dish, one per droplet.
4. *Orientation and dissection:* Using the holding pipette, orient the embryo to avoid blastomere damage. Pass the injection pipette through the ZP on one side and again on the opposing side.
5. *Tearing:* Move the embryo along the injection pipette and rub the ZP between the injection and holding pipettes until it tears. Repeat to create a V-shaped flap if necessary.

Zona Drilling by Laser

Laser-assisted zona drilling uses contact or noncontact lasers to create an opening in the ZP. The procedure involves the following steps:

1. *Laser types:* Both ultraviolet and infrared spectrum lasers can be used. Noncontact lasers, especially those operating in the infrared spectrum, are preferred due to reduced risk of damage to surrounding tissues.
2. *Procedure:* Align the ZP to be drilled and fire the laser to create a hole or slit. The size of the opening is controlled by the laser's power and duration.
3. *Precision:* Drill successive small holes if necessary, rather than attempting to breach the ZP with a single shot, to avoid damage to the oocyte or blastomeres.

CONCLUSION

Assisted hatching is a significant advancement in ART, providing increased implantation potential for certain patient groups. The technique, when performed with precision, can enhance the chances of successful pregnancy, particularly in women of advanced maternal age, those with repeated IVF failures, and embryos with thick or hardened ZP. The choice of technique—whether mechanical, chemical, laser, or piezo technology—should be tailored to the individual patient's needs to ensure optimal outcomes.[8]

REFERENCES

1. Schoolcraft WB, Schlenker T, Gee M, Stevens J, Sahakian V. Assisted hatching in women ≥38 years of age. Fertil Steril. 1999;72(4):603-6.
2. Balaban B, Urman B, Sertac A, Alatas C, Aksoy S, Mercan R. A randomized controlled study of assisted hatching in patients undergoing IVF. Hum Reprod. 2002;17(6):1848-52.
3. Rienzi L, Ubaldi F, Anniballo R, Greco E. Assisted hatching in human reproduction: a review. Hum Reprod Update. 2002;8(6):686-95.
4. Cohen J, Alikani M, Trowbridge J, Rosenwaks Z. Implantation enhancement by selective assisted hatching using zona drilling of human embryos with poor prognosis. Hum Reprod. 1992;7(5):685-91.
5. Malter HE, Cohen J. Blastocyst formation and hatching in vitro following zona drilling of mouse and human embryos. Gamete Res. 1989;24(1):67-80.
6. Antinori S, Versaci C, Dani G, Selman H, Colpi G, Levi-Setti P, Cittadini E. Laser-assisted hatching of human embryos prior to implantation: a preliminary report. Hum Reprod. 1996;11(1):149-154.
7. Sallam HN, Sadek SS, Agameya AF. Assisted hatching—a meta-analysis of randomized controlled trials. J Assist Reprod Genet. 2003;20(8):332-42.
8. Tadir Y, Wright WH, Vafa O, Ord T, Asch RH, Berns MW. Piezo micromanipulation for assisted hatching of human embryos. J In Vitro Fertil Embryo Transf. 1993;10(3):139-44.

CHAPTER 16

Embryo Biopsy and Preimplantation Genetic Diagnosis

INTRODUCTION

Embryo biopsy is a groundbreaking procedure in assisted reproductive technology (ART) that allows for the genetic evaluation of embryos before implantation. It plays a pivotal role in preimplantation genetic testing (PGT), enabling the identification of genetic abnormalities and improving the likelihood of successful pregnancy outcomes. Conducted at either the cleavage stage (day 3) or the blastocyst stage (day 5), embryo biopsy techniques have evolved to balance precision with embryo viability. This chapter delves into the methodologies, advantages, and challenges of blastomere and blastocyst biopsy, shedding light on their critical role in enhancing the effectiveness of ART and facilitating informed decision-making for couples undergoing treatment.

INTRODUCTION TO EMBRYO BIOPSY

Embryo biopsy is a critical procedure in preimplantation genetic testing (PGT), allowing for the genetic analysis of embryos before their transfer in assisted reproductive technology (ART). The two primary stages at which embryo biopsy can be performed are the cleavage stage (day 3) and the blastocyst stage (day 5) **(Table 1)**. Each stage has its specific techniques, advantages, and challenges. This chapter provides a detailed overview of both blastomere biopsy on day 3 and blastocyst biopsy on day 5, including the steps involved in each procedure.

BLASTOMERE BIOPSY

Overview

Blastomere biopsy is performed on embryos at the cleavage stage, typically on day 3 of

TABLE 1: Comparison of day-3 and day-5 biopsies.

Criteria	*Day-3 biopsy*	*Day-5 biopsy*
Genetic analysis	Limited to one or two cells, potentially leading to higher diagnostic errors due to mosaicism[1]	Multiple trophectoderm (TE) cells provide a more accurate and comprehensive genetic profile, reducing the risk of mosaicism-related diagnostic errors[7]
Embryo viability	Higher risk of compromising embryo viability due to removal of blastomeres critical for early development[1]	Lower risk of affecting the embryo's viability as only TE cells are removed, preserving the inner cell mass (ICM)[7]
Timing and logistics	Allows for fresh embryo transfer within the same cycle after genetic results[4]	Often requires cryopreservation of embryos and transfer in a subsequent cycle, potentially delaying the process[7]

development when the embryo consists of around 6–8 cells. This technique involves the removal of one or two blastomeres (cells) from the embryo for genetic analysis.[1]

Steps Involved in Blastomere Biopsy

1. *Embryo preparation:* On day 3, embryos are evaluated for quality and development. Suitable embryos (6–8 cells with minimal fragmentation) are selected for biopsy.[1]
2. *Zona pellucida (ZP) breaching:* The ZP, the protective outer layer of the embryo, is breached using one of the following methods:
   a. *Laser drilling:* A precise laser is used to create a small hole in the ZP.[2]
   b. *Chemical drilling:* Acid Tyrode's solution is applied to dissolve a part of the ZP.[3]
   c. *Mechanical drilling:* A micropipette is used to physically puncture the ZP.[3]
3. *Blastomere removal:*
   a. A holding pipette stabilizes the embryo **(Figs. 1 and 2)**.
   b. A biopsy pipette is carefully inserted through the opening in the ZP to aspirate one or two blastomeres **(Figs. 3 and 4)**.

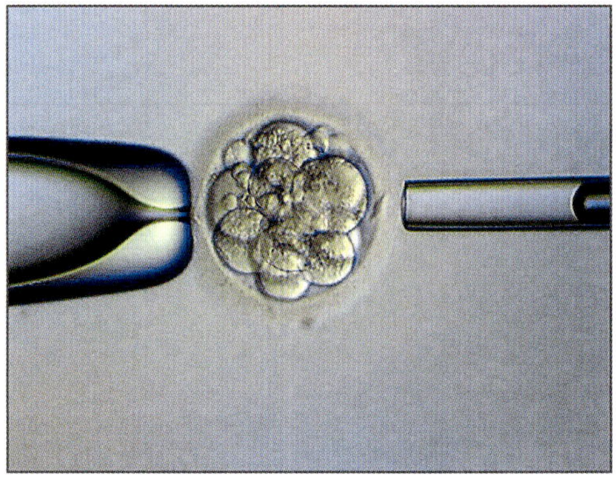

Fig. 2: Position the embryo so that the desired blastomere for biopsy is easily accessible.

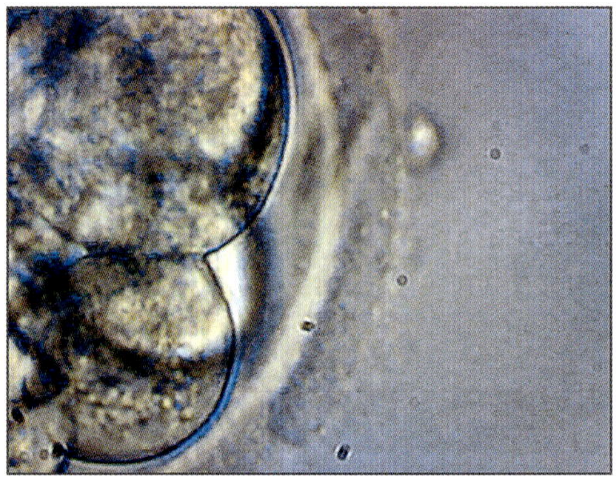

Fig. 3: Use a laser to thin the zona and create an appropriately sized hole to allow the needle to easily penetrate the zona.

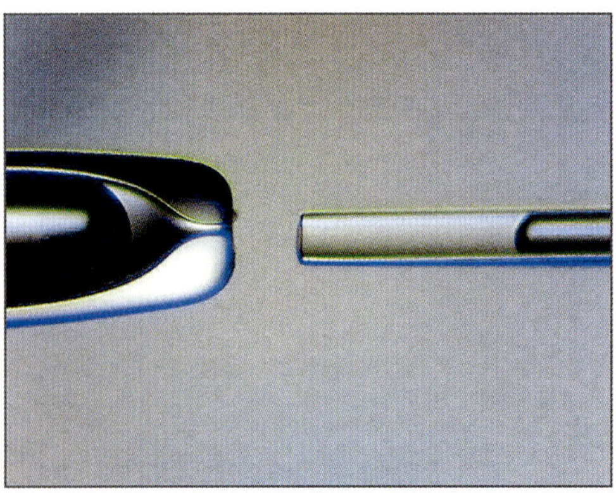

Fig. 1: The holding pipette and biopsy pipette are aligned and rinsed in culture media.

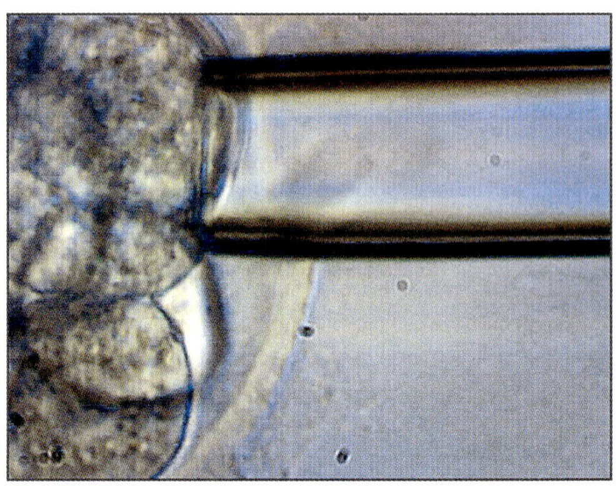

Fig. 4: Gently aspirate the blastomere intended for biopsy.

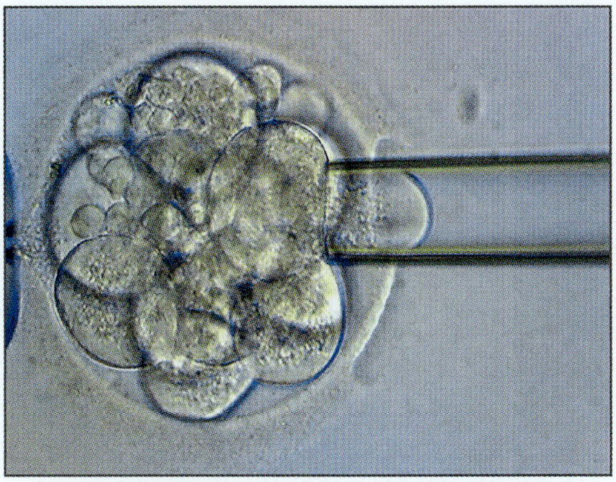

Fig. 5: Gently remove the blastomere.

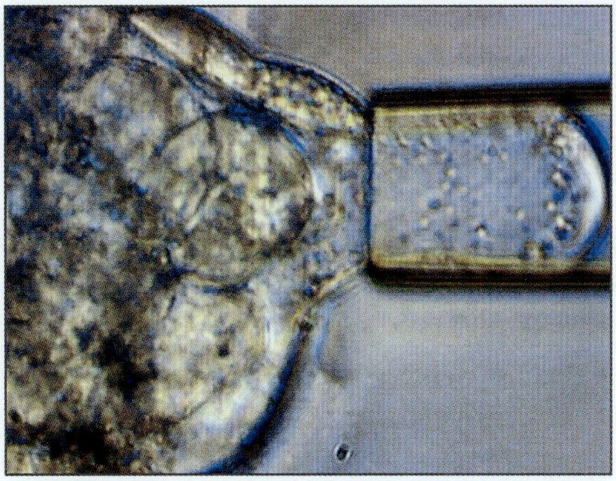

Fig. 6: For a day-5 biopsy, position the embryo away from the inner cell mass (ICM), and use the biopsy pipette to aspirate the trophectoderm (TE) cells. Use a laser to separate the cells.

   c. Care is taken to avoid damaging the remaining cells and to ensure the biopsied cells are viable for genetic analysis **(Fig. 5)**.[1]
4. *Embryo culture:* After biopsy, embryos are returned to the culture medium and incubated until the results of the genetic tests are available or frozen on day 5.[4]
5. *Genetic analysis:* The removed blastomeres are subjected to genetic analysis using techniques such as fluorescence in situ hybridization (FISH), polymerase chain reaction (PCR), or next-generation sequencing (NGS).[5]

Advantages and Disadvantages

- *Advantages:* It allows for early detection of genetic abnormalities and provides time for comprehensive genetic analysis before embryo transfer.[6]
- *Disadvantage:* The removal of blastomeres can potentially impact the embryo's developmental potential and viability.[1]

BLASTOCYST BIOPSY

Overview

Blastocyst biopsy is performed on embryos at the blastocyst stage, typically on day 5 or 6 of development when the embryo has differentiated into the inner cell mass (ICM) and the trophectoderm (TE). This technique involves the removal of several TE cells, which are destined to form the placenta.[7]

Steps Involved in Blastocyst Biopsy

1. *Embryo preparation:* On day 5 or 6, embryos are assessed for quality and development. Blastocysts with a well-defined ICM and TE are selected for biopsy.[7]
2. *Zona pellucida breaching:* A laser is typically used to create a hole in the ZP to facilitate the biopsy.[7]
3. *TE cell removal:*
   a. The blastocyst is held in place using a holding pipette.
   b. A laser is used to facilitate the detachment of several TE cells from the blastocyst.
   c. A biopsy pipette is then used to aspirate these TE cells, ensuring minimal disruption to the ICM **(Fig. 6)**.[7]
4. *Embryo culture:* Post biopsy, blastocysts are cultured for a short period to monitor their continued development and ensure they remain viable and are then frozen until results arrive.[8]

5. *Genetic analysis:* The TE cells are subjected to genetic analysis using advanced techniques like NGS, which provides comprehensive chromosomal information.[5]

Advantages and Disadvantages

- *Advantages:* More cells can be biopsied at this stage, increasing the accuracy of genetic testing. The procedure is less likely to affect the viability of the embryo as the cells removed are from the TE, not the ICM, which will form the fetus.[7]
- *Disadvantage:* Later-stage biopsy means less time for genetic analysis before transfer, potentially necessitating embryo freezing and later transfer cycles.[9]

Both day-3 blastomere biopsy and day-5 blastocyst biopsy are valuable techniques in ART for PGT. The choice of method depends on various factors, including the patient's specific circumstances, the quality and development stage of the embryos, and the specific goals of genetic testing. Careful consideration and expertise are required to perform these biopsies effectively, ensuring minimal harm to the embryos while providing accurate genetic information to inform treatment decisions.

Technical Considerations and Best Practices

- *Embryo handling:* Embryos should be handled minimally and maintained in a stable environment to reduce stress and potential damage.[10]
- *Micromanipulation skills:* Proficiency in micromanipulation is crucial for performing precise biopsies. Training and experience are essential to prevent damage to the embryo.[7]
- *Laser versus mechanical methods:* Laser-assisted hatching is generally preferred for its precision and reduced mechanical stress on embryos. However, both methods are effective when performed correctly.[9]
- *Cell number and quality:* Adequate cell sampling without compromising embryo viability is critical. Typically, 5–10 TE cells are sufficient for reliable genetic analysis.[11]

PREIMPLANTATION GENETIC DIAGNOSIS AND PREIMPLANTATION GENETIC SCREENING TECHNIQUES

Overview of Genetic Screening Techniques

Preimplantation genetic diagnosis (PGD) and preimplantation genetic screening (PGS) are advanced techniques used to detect genetic abnormalities in embryos before implantation **(Table 2)**.

- *PGD:* PGD is used to identify specific genetic disorders in embryos, typically those known to affect one or both parents. It allows for the selection of embryos free from these genetic conditions.[12]
    - *PGS*: PGS screens embryos for aneuploidy, which refers to an abnormal number of chromosomes. This screening helps identify embryos with the highest likelihood of successful implantation and healthy development.[13]

Technological Advances

- *NGS:* NGS has revolutionized PGD and PGS by providing more accurate and comprehensive genetic analyses. It allows for the detection of smaller chromosomal abnormalities and single-gene defects with high precision.[11]
- *Array comparative genomic hybridization (aCGH):* This technique enables the analysis of all 24 chromosomes simultaneously, enhancing the detection of

TABLE 2: Clinical indications and benefits.

Criteria	*Preimplantation genetic diagnosis (PGD)*	*Preimplantation genetic screening (PGS)*
Indications	This is indicated for couples at risk of transmitting single-gene disorders (e.g., cystic fibrosis, Huntington's disease, thalassemia), chromosomal translocations, and other inherited genetic abnormalities	This is recommended for older women (typically over 35 years), couples with recurrent pregnancy loss, repeated in vitro fertilization (IVF) failures, and male factor infertility (e.g., severe oligospermia, azoospermia)
Benefits	It allows couples to prevent the transmission of genetic disorders, reducing the emotional and financial burden postnatally. It increases the likelihood of a successful pregnancy with a genetically healthy embryo	It improves implantation rates, reduces miscarriage risk, and increases the chances of delivering a healthy baby. By identifying euploid embryos, PGS enhances overall IVF success rates
Testing method	It focuses on specific genetic mutations or chromosomal abnormalities. It typically involves biopsying one or more cells from an early-stage embryo	It screens all 23 chromosome pairs in embryos to identify aneuploidies, improving selection of embryos with the normal chromosomal number
Target population	Couples with known genetic conditions or history of inherited disorders; especially useful for those with known carrier status for specific genetic mutations	Couples with no known genetic conditions but higher risk factors like advanced maternal age, repeated IVF failure, or unexplained infertility
Limitations	Limited to specific known genetic issues, not useful for detecting all chromosomal abnormalities; may miss mosaicism depending on the stage of biopsy	It does not diagnose specific genetic disorders but rather identifies chromosomal abnormalities. It may still miss low-level mosaicism or some structural chromosomal rearrangements
Clinical outcomes	It primarily prevents the birth of a child with a specific genetic disorder, significantly reducing disease burden in affected families	It increases the overall success rate of IVF by improving embryo selection, leading to higher live birth rates and lower miscarriage rates
Procedure timing	Typically performed on day-3 or day-5 embryos, depending on the method of biopsy used	Usually performed on day-5 blastocysts, allowing for more accurate screening due to a larger sample size

aneuploidies and structural chromosomal abnormalities.[6]

CONCLUSION

Embryo biopsy coupled with PGD and PGS offers significant advantages in ART by enabling the selection of genetically healthy embryos, thus improving implantation rates, reducing miscarriages, and ensuring the birth of healthy babies.

REFERENCES

1. Hardarson T, et al. Preimplantation genetic screening in women of advanced maternal age decreases implantation rate without affecting live birth rate. Reprod Biomed Online . 2008;17(6):641-6.
2. De Vos A, Van Steirteghem A. Zona hardening, zona drilling and assisted hatching. Reprod Biomed Online . 2000;2(1):24-8.
3. Cohen J, Alikani M, Trowbridge J, Rosenwaks Z. Implantation enhancement by selective

assisted hatching using zona drilling of human embryos with poor prognosis. Hum Reprod. 1992;7(5):685-91.
4. Harper JC, Harton G. The use of arrays in preimplantation genetic diagnosis and screening. Fertil Steril. 2010;94(4): 1173-7.
5. Mastenbroek S, et al. In vitro fertilization with preimplantation genetic screening. SEN Engl J Med. 2011; 357(1):9-17.
6. Harper JC, Sengupta SB. Preimplantation genetic diagnosis: state of the art 2011. Human Genet. 2012;131(2):175-86.
7. Scott RT, et al. Comprehensive chromosome screening is highly predictive of the reproductive potential of human embryos: A prospective, blinded, nonselection study. Fertil Steril. 2013;100(2):408-13.
8. Schoolcraft WB, Treff NR, Stevens JM, Ferry K, Katz-Jaffe M, Scott RT Jr. Live birth outcome with trophectoderm biopsy, blastocyst vitrification, and single-nucleotide polymorphism microarray-based comprehensive chromosome screening in infertile patients. Fertil Steril. 2011;96(3):638-40.
9. Harper JC, et al. The ESHRE PGD Consortium: 10 years of data collection. Hum Reprod Update. 2010;16(2):234-47.
10. Thornhill AR, deDie-Smulders CE, Geraedts JP, Harper JC, Harton GL, Lavery SA, et al.; ESHRE PGD Consortium. ESHRE PGD Consortium 'Best practice guidelines for organization of a PGD centre for PGD/ preimplantation genetic screening (PGS)'. Hum Reprod. 2005;20(1):35-48.
11. Capalbo A, Bono S, Spizzichino L, Biricik A, Baldi M, Colamaria S, et al. Sequential comprehensive chromosome analysis on polar bodies, blastomeres and trophoblast: Insights into female meiotic errors and chromosomal segregation in the preimplantation window of embryo development. Hum Reprod. 2013;28(2): 509-18.
12. Kuliev A, et al. Preimplantation genetic diagnosis for hemophilia. J Assist Reprod Genet. 2011;28(2):125-9.
13. Munné S, Sandalinas M, Escudero T, Velilla E, Walmsley R, Sadowy S, et al. Improved implantation after preimplantation genetic diagnosis of aneuploidy. Reprod Biomed Online. 2003;7(1):91-7.

17 CHAPTER

Vitrification and Thawing of Oocytes and Embryos

INTRODUCTION

Vitrification is a transformative cryopreservation technique in assisted reproductive technology (ART), offering superior outcomes compared to traditional slow freezing methods. This process rapidly cools oocytes and embryos to a glass-like state, preventing ice crystal formation that can damage cellular structures. With significantly higher survival rates and post-thaw viability, vitrification has become the gold standard for preserving reproductive cells. The technique provides flexibility for fertility preservation, enabling patients to store oocytes or embryos for future use, particularly beneficial for those undergoing medical treatments or planning to delay childbearing. Vitrification has revolutionized ART by improving clinical outcomes and expanding options for reproductive preservation.

PRINCIPLES OF VITRIFICATION

Advantages over Traditional Cryopreservation

Vitrification is a pivotal cryopreservation technique in assisted reproductive technology (ART) that has revolutionized the preservation of oocytes and embryos. Unlike traditional slow freezing methods, which often result in the formation of ice crystals that can damage delicate cellular structures, vitrification involves the rapid cooling of biological samples to a glass-like state.[1] This ultrarapid cooling process, combined with the use of high concentrations of cryoprotectants, effectively prevents ice crystal formation, thereby minimizing the risk of cellular damage.

One of the key advantages of vitrification is its ability to significantly improve the survival rates of oocytes and embryos after thawing. The process reduces cryoinjury—damage that cells can experience during freezing—by maintaining the structural integrity and functionality of the preserved cells. As a result, vitrified oocytes and embryos often demonstrate similar, if not superior, implantation and pregnancy outcomes compared to those achieved with fresh specimens.[2] This has made vitrification the method of choice for cryopreservation in many ART laboratories.

Advantages of vitrification:

- *Higher survival rates:* Vitrification significantly improves the survival rates of oocytes and embryos compared to traditional slow freezing. This is due to the elimination of ice crystal formation, which can cause cellular injury.[2]
- *Increased post-thaw viability:* The rapid cooling and solidification of cellular contents help maintain the integrity of cell membranes and organelles. As a result, oocytes and embryos vitrified using this method show higher post-thaw viability and developmental potential.[1]

- *Enhanced clinical outcomes:* Numerous studies have reported improved clinical outcomes, including higher implantation and pregnancy rates, with vitrified oocytes and embryos. The success of vitrification has made it the preferred method in many IVF clinics.[3]
- *Flexibility and convenience:* Vitrification allows for the flexible scheduling of embryo transfers and facilitates the banking of oocytes and embryos for future use. This flexibility is particularly beneficial for patients undergoing fertility preservation before medical treatments such as chemotherapy.[4]

Step-by-Step Vitrification Protocol

The vitrification process involves several critical steps to ensure the successful preservation of oocytes and embryos. The protocol typically includes the following stages:

1. *Preparation of solutions:* Three solutions are prepared: A (i) base solution (BS), an (ii) equilibration solution (ES) and a (iii) vitrification solution (VS) **(Table 1)**. The ES contains a lower concentration of cryoprotectants, while the VS has a higher concentration to induce rapid dehydration and vitrification.[2]
2. *Equilibration:* Oocytes or embryos are first placed in the ES to allow gradual dehydration and to prevent osmotic shock. This step typically lasts for 5–10 minutes, depending on the developmental stage of the oocytes or embryos.[3]
3. *Vitrification:* After equilibration, the samples are quickly transferred to the VS. This solution induces rapid dehydration and vitrification within seconds. The samples are then loaded onto specialized carriers, such as Cryotop or VitriFit, which facilitate ultrarapid cooling.[2]
4. *Immediate cooling:* The carriers with the vitrified samples are immediately plunged into liquid nitrogen (LN_2) to achieve rapid cooling and solidification. This step is critical to prevent ice crystal formation and ensure successful vitrification.[1]
5. *Storage:* The vitrified samples are stored in LN_2 at –196°C until they are needed for thawing and use in ART procedures.[4]

TABLE 1: Vitrification solutions.

Solution	*Description*	*Components*
Base solution (BS)	It is the initial solution used to begin dehydration and equilibration of oocytes/embryos	• Base culture medium (e.g., MOPS, HEPES) • Balanced salt solution (e.g., PBS, HTF) • Supplemented with proteins (e.g., serum albumin)
Equilibration solution (ES)	It is used to gradually replace water with cryoprotectants, allowing cells to equilibrate	• BS • 7.5–15% ethylene glycol (EG) • 7.5–15% dimethyl sulphoxide (DMSO) • Protein supplement (e.g., serum albumin)
Vitrification solution (VS)	It is a highly concentrated cryoprotectant solution used for rapid cooling and vitrification	• BS • 15–20% EG • 15–20% DMSO • 0.5–1.0 M sucrose • Protein supplement (e.g., serum albumin)

(HTF: human tubal fluid; PBS: phosphate buffered saline)

THAWING PROTOCOLS

Optimizing Survival Rates during Thawing

The thawing process is as crucial as the vitrification process, requiring careful execution to maximize survival rates and maintain the viability of oocytes and embryos.

- *Preparation of warming solutions:* Three warming solutions are prepared—(1) thawing solution (TS), (2) dilution solution (DS), and (3) washing solution (WS) **(Table 2)**. These solutions vary in cryoprotectant concentration, with TS having a high concentration for immediate rehydration, while DS and WS gradually reduce cryoprotectants to prevent osmotic shock.[3]
- *Initial thawing:* The vitrified oocytes or embryos are first immersed in TS at 37°C. This step lasts approximately 1 minute, allowing rapid rehydration while preventing ice crystal formation as the samples warm up.[2]
- *Stepwise rehydration:* After the initial thaw, the oocytes or embryos are transferred sequentially to DS and WS. Each step lasts for 3–5 minutes, facilitating gradual removal of cryoprotectants while ensuring controlled rehydration of the cells.[2]
- *Washing:* Following rehydration, the oocytes or embryos are washed in a series of pre-equilibrated culture media to further remove any residual cryoprotectants. This step is crucial for restoring the physiological environment for post-thaw recovery.
- *Incubation:* The thawed oocytes or embryos are incubated in culture media at 37°C with 5% CO_2 to recover from the thawing process. They remain in the incubator for a period of 2–4 hours before being assessed for survival and further use in ART procedures.

POST-THAW ASSESSMENT AND HANDLING

After thawing, it is essential to assess the viability and quality of the oocytes or embryos before proceeding with ART procedures.

- *Morphological assessment:* The first step in post-thaw assessment is a thorough morphological examination. This involves checking for any signs of damage, such as membrane integrity, cytoplasmic granularity, and overall cell structure.[3]
- *Viability testing:* In some cases, viability testing, such as staining with vital

TABLE 2: Thawing solutions.

Solution	*Description*	*Components*
Thawing solution (TS)	The initial solution is used to rapidly warm vitrified oocytes/embryos	• Base culture medium • 1.0 M sucrose • Protein supplement (e.g., serum albumin)
Dilution solution (DS)	It is used to gradually remove cryoprotectants and rehydrate cells	• Base culture medium • 0.5 M sucrose • Protein supplement (e.g., serum albumin)
Washing solution (WS)	It is used to wash away residual cryoprotectants and prepare oocytes/embryos for culture	• Base culture medium • 0.25 M sucrose • Protein supplement (e.g., serum albumin)

TABLE 3: Key points on fertility preservation.

Aspect	*Scientific points*
Cryopreservation techniques	Vitrification is the preferred method for preserving oocytes and embryos due to its high survival rates and minimized cryoinjury
Oocyte preservation	Vital for women wishing to delay childbearing for personal, medical, or professional reasons; it involves the retrieval and vitrification of oocytes
Embryo preservation	It is ideal for couples undergoing IVF who may want to store embryos for future use, allowing flexibility in family planning
Sperm preservation	Sperm can be frozen for men undergoing medical treatments or for those who may face occupational hazards affecting fertility
Ovarian tissue cryopreservation	It is an experimental technique used to preserve ovarian tissue, which can later be reimplanted to restore fertility or hormonal function
Preimplantation genetic testing (PGT)	Vitrified embryos can be biopsied for genetic testing, ensuring only healthy embryos are implanted while preserving reproductive potential
Long-term storage	Cryopreserved oocytes, sperm, and embryos can be stored for extended periods, retaining their viability and developmental potential upon thawing
Ethical considerations	It involves decisions about the future use, donation, or disposal of stored reproductive material, with respect to patients' autonomy and preferences
Legal and regulatory aspects	Fertility preservation is governed by laws and guidelines that vary by country, ensuring the ethical handling, consent, and use of preserved reproductive cells

dyes, can be performed to confirm the functional integrity of the thawed oocytes or embryos.[2]

- *Culture and monitoring:* Thawed embryos are typically cultured for a short period to monitor their development before transfer. This step allows for the identification of any delayed damage and ensures that only viable embryos are selected for transfer.[1]
- *Handling:* Gentle handling and minimal exposure to suboptimal conditions are crucial during the post-thaw process to maintain the viability and developmental potential of the oocytes or embryos.[4]

Fertility Preservation

Fertility preservation involves the use of cryopreservation techniques to safeguard reproductive potential in individuals facing medical treatments or conditions that may impair fertility **(Table 3)**. Oocyte, embryo, and gonadal tissue cryopreservation are the most commonly employed methods. These techniques are essential for patients undergoing chemotherapy, radiation, or other treatments that may damage reproductive cells, allowing them the possibility of future reproduction once treatment is complete.

CONCLUSION

Vitrification and thawing represent groundbreaking advancements in the field of ART, fundamentally transforming how oocytes and embryos are preserved and utilized. These sophisticated techniques have elevated the standards of fertility treatments by offering more reliable and effective options for preserving reproductive cells, which is crucial for both current and future family-building efforts. The ability to successfully vitrify and thaw oocytes and embryos with high survival and developmental rates has not only improved clinical outcomes but also expanded the possibilities for patients who may need to delay childbearing or preserve fertility due to medical treatments.

REFERENCES

1. Al-Inany H, Youssef MA, Ayeleke RO, Brown J, Lam WS, Broekmans FJ. Vitrification versus slow freezing for women undergoing oocyte cryopreservation. Cochrane Database Syst Rev. 2016;2016(8):CD010047.
2. Kuwayama M, Vajta G, Kato O, Leibo SP. Highly efficient vitrification method for cryopreservation of human oocytes. Reprod Biomed Online. 2005;11(3):300-8.
3. Rienzi L, Romano S, Albricci L, Maggiulli R, Capalbo A, Baroni E, et al. Embryo development of fresh 'versus' vitrified metaphase II oocytes after ICSI: a prospective randomized sibling-oocyte study. Hum Reprod. 2010; 25(1):66-73.
4. Cobo A, Kuwayama M, Pérez S, Ruiz A, Pellicer A, Remohí J. Comparison of concomitant outcome achieved with fresh and cryopreserved donor oocytes vitrified by the cryotop method. Fertil Steril. 2008; 89(6): 1657-64.

18 CHAPTER

Ethical and Legal Considerations in Assisted Reproductive Technology

INTRODUCTION

Ethical and legal considerations in assisted reproductive technology (ART) are essential to ensure the well-being of all parties involved, including patients, donors, surrogates, and offspring. Central to these considerations are robust record-keeping practices, informed consent, and patient confidentiality, which uphold transparency, trust, and compliance with regulatory standards. Additionally, the use of donor gametes and surrogacy introduces complex ethical dilemmas and legal requirements, such as maintaining donor anonymity and defining parental rights. Laws like India's Assisted Reproductive Technology (Regulation) Act, 2021, and Surrogacy (Regulation) Act, 2021, provide a structured framework to guide ART practices, emphasizing ethical standards and the protection of patient rights while addressing advances in reproductive technology.

RECORD KEEPING AND MAINTAINING LOGS

Importance of Record Keeping in ART

Effective record keeping in assisted reproductive technology (ART) is crucial for ensuring high standards of care, compliance with legal and regulatory requirements, and the facilitation of research and quality control. Comprehensive and accurate records are essential for tracking the treatment and outcomes of each patient, monitoring laboratory procedures, and ensuring traceability of all materials used in the ART process.[1]

COMPONENTS OF ART RECORDS

Key components of ART records include:

- *Patient information:* Detailed medical histories, consent forms, and treatment plans for each patient
- *Laboratory logs:* Documentation of all laboratory procedures, including gamete and embryo handling, culture conditions, quality control and cryopreservation details
- *Treatment outcomes:* Records of fertilization rates, embryo quality assessments, implantation outcomes, and pregnancy results
- *Equipment maintenance:* Logs of maintenance and calibration of laboratory equipment to ensure optimal functioning and compliance with regulatory standards[2]

PATIENT CONSENTS

Informed Consent in ART

Obtaining informed consent from patients undergoing ART is a fundamental ethical and legal requirement. Informed consent ensures that patients are fully aware of the nature of the treatment, potential risks, benefits, and alternatives, allowing them to make educated decisions about their care.[3]

TABLE 1: Maintenance of consent forms in assisted reproductive technology (ART) clinics and banks in India.

Category	Description	Form number
Level 1/level 2 ART clinics	Consent form to be signed by the couple or woman	Form 6
	Consent for intrauterine insemination (IUI) with husband's semen or sperm	Form 7
	Consent for IUI with donor semen	Form 8
	Consent for freezing of embryos	Form 9
	Consent for freezing gametes	Form 10
	Assent for freezing of gametes (sperm or oocytes) and parental consent	Form 11
	Consent for oocyte retrieval	Form 12
	Consent from oocyte donor	Form 13
ART banks	Record of use of donor gametes	Forms 14, 14A, and 14B
	Consent form for the donor of sperm	Form 15

Elements of Informed Consent

- *Disclosure:* Providing detailed information about the ART procedures, including the steps involved, success rates, potential risks, and alternatives
- *Comprehension:* Ensuring that patients understand the information provided, often through discussions and providing written materials
- *Voluntariness:* Confirming that the decision to proceed with ART is made freely, without coercion or undue influence
- *Documentation:* Properly documenting the consent process, including signed consent forms and records of discussions **(Table 1)**[4]

CONFIDENTIALITY AND ANONYMITY

Ensuring Patient Confidentiality

Confidentiality is a cornerstone of patient trust in medical practice, including ART. Ensuring the confidentiality of patient information involves implementing robust data protection measures, restricting access to patient records, and complying with relevant privacy laws and regulations.[5]

Maintaining Anonymity in Donor Programs

Anonymity in gamete donation programs protects the identities of both donors and recipients. This involves coding systems to ensure that identifying information is not disclosed, and strict protocols for handling and storing donor information.[6] However, evolving regulations and societal views on donor anonymity are leading to more open practices in some regions worldwide.

Legal and Ethical Considerations

The use of donor gametes in ART raises significant legal and ethical issues, including the rights and responsibilities of donors, recipients, and offspring. Regulations often specify criteria for donor selection, screening, and compensation, as well as the rights of donor-conceived individuals to access information about their genetic origins.[7]

THE ASSISTED REPRODUCTIVE TECHNOLOGY (REGULATION) ACT, 2021—INDIA

India's Assisted Reproductive Technology (Regulation) Act, 2021, provides a comprehensive framework for the regulation of ART services, including the use of donor gametes. Key provisions include:

- *Eligibility criteria:* Clear guidelines on the eligibility of donors, including age limits, medical and genetic screening, and psychological evaluation
- *Staff eligibility:* Clear and defined criteria for staff eligibility, including necessary qualifications, certifications, and relevant experience in ART, along with ongoing training to ensure competency in handling gametes, embryos, and patient care **(Table 2)**
- *Equipment requirement:* All equipment used in ART laboratories must meet rigorous standards for precision, sterility, and calibration, including incubators, microscopes, and cryopreservation systems, ensuring optimal conditions for handling and culturing gametes, embryos, and other biological materials **(Table 3)**.
- *Consent:* Mandatory informed consent from donors, ensuring they understand the implications and potential future use of their gametes
- *Confidentiality:* Strict confidentiality protocols to protect the identities of donors and recipients
- *Compensation:* Regulations on the permissible compensation for donors to prevent exploitation and ensure ethical practices[8]

SURROGACY

Ethical and Legal Frameworks

Surrogacy involves complex ethical and legal considerations, particularly regarding the rights and responsibilities of the surrogate, intended parents, and the child. Legal frameworks vary widely across different jurisdictions, addressing issues such as the enforceability of surrogacy agreements, parental rights, and the welfare of the child.[9]

The Surrogacy (Regulation) Act, 2021—India

India's Surrogacy (Regulation) Act, 2021, aims to regulate surrogacy practices to ensure ethical standards and protect the interests of all parties involved. The key provisions include:

- *Staff eligibility:* Staff involved in surrogacy must meet strict eligibility criteria, including appropriate qualifications, certifications, and experience. Ongoing training is essential to ensure competency in handling biological materials and patient care **(Table 4)**.
- *Eligibility of intended parents:* Criteria for intended parents, including marital status, age, and medical necessity for surrogacy
- *Surrogate eligibility:* Requirements for surrogates, such as age limits, previous experience with childbirth, and medical fitness
- *Altruistic surrogacy:* Prohibition of commercial surrogacy, allowing only altruistic surrogacy where the surrogate receives no financial compensation beyond medical expenses and insurance coverage
- *Consent:* Informed consent from all parties, including the surrogate and intended parents, is mandatory. This ensures that they fully understand the legal, medical, and ethical implications of surrogacy, including the transfer of legal parentage and the use of any reproductive materials **(Table 5)**.

TABLE 2: Staff requirements and qualifications in ART clinics and banks in India.

Staff position	***ART clinic level***	***Requirements***	***Qualifications***
Gynecologist	ART level 1	Minimum 01 gynecologist	Medical postgraduate in gynecology and obstetrics
Gynecologist	ART level 2	Minimum 01 gynecologist	*Medical postgraduate in gynecology and obstetrics with:* • Record of performing 50 ovum pickup procedures under supervision of a trained ART specialist • At least 3 years of working experience in an ART clinic, OR Medical postgraduate in gynecology and obstetrics with super specialist Doctorate of Medicine or fellowship in reproductive medicine with at least 3 years of working experience in an ART clinic
Anesthetist	ART level 2	Minimum 01 anesthetist	Medical postgraduate in anesthesia
Embryologist	ART level 2	Minimum 01 embryologist	Postgraduate in clinical embryology with at least 3 years of human ART laboratory experience, OR PhD in clinical embryology OR related field with at least 1 year of human ART laboratory experience, OR Medical graduate (MBBS) or Veterinary graduate (BVSc) with a postgraduate degree in Clinical Embryology with at least 2 years of human ART laboratory experience, OR postgraduate in Life Sciences or Biotechnology with at least 1 year of certified clinical embryology training and 4 years' experience in an ART laboratory
Counselor	ART level 2	Minimum 01 counselor	Graduate in Psychology, Clinical Psychology, Nursing, or Life Sciences
Director	ART level 2	Minimum 01 director	Postgraduate degree in Medical or Life Sciences or Management Sciences
Andrologist	ART level 2	Optional	MCh or DNB in Urology with special training in diagnosing and treating male infertility
Registered Medical Practitioner	ART bank	Minimum 01 Registered Medical Practitioner trained in handling, preparation, and storage of semen samples	Trained in the handling, preparation, and storage of semen samples

TABLE 3: Minimum equipment in ART clinics and banks in India.

Category	Equipment
ART level 1 clinics	• Microscope • Centrifuge • Refrigerator
ART level 2 clinics	• Microscope • Incubator (minimum 02 in number) • Laminar airflow • Sperm counting chambers • Centrifuge • Refrigerator • Equipment for cryopreservation • Ovum aspiration pump • Ultrasonography (USG) machine with transvaginal probe and needle guard • Test tube warmer • Anesthesia resuscitation trolley
ART banks	• Centrifuge machine • Incubator • Microscope • Laminar air flow

TABLE 4: Staff requirement and qualification for surrogacy clinics.

Staff position	Requirements	Qualifications
Gynecologist	Minimum 01 gynecologist	Medical postgraduate in gynecology and obstetrics with at least 3 years of experience in an ART clinic and a record of performing 50 ovum pickups
Andrologist	Optional	Master of Chirurgiae or Diplomate of National Board in urology with special training in diagnosing and treating male infertility
Embryologist	Minimum 01 embryologist	Postgraduate in clinical embryology with at least 3 years of experience in handling human gametes and embryos, or a PhD in Clinical Embryology/ART with additional 1 year experience
Counselor	Minimum 01 counselor	Graduate in psychology, clinical psychology, nursing, or life sciences from a recognized university
Anesthetist	Minimum 01 anesthetist	Medical postgraduate in Anesthesia from a recognized university

- *Legal parentage:* Clear guidelines on the transfer of legal parentage from the surrogate to the intended parents, ensuring the child's legal status and rights are secure[10]

CONCLUSION

The practice of ART involves navigating complex ethical and legal landscapes to ensure the welfare and rights of all involved parties. Comprehensive record keeping,

TABLE 5: Forms to be maintained by surrogacy clinics.

Form number	***Purpose***
Form 1	Application form for couple of Indian origin/intending woman for availing surrogacy addressed to board
Form 2	Consent of the surrogate mother and agreement for surrogacy
Form 3	Application form for registration of a surrogacy clinic
Form 4	Certificate of registration for a surrogacy clinic
Form 5	Appeal form against the order passed by the appropriate authority

obtaining informed consent, maintaining confidentiality and anonymity, and adhering to regulations concerning donor gametes and surrogacy are essential to uphold ethical standards and legal compliance. The Assisted Reproductive Technology (Regulation) Act, 2021 and the Surrogacy (Regulation) Act, 2021 in India provide a robust framework to regulate and guide ART practices, reflecting the latest advancements and ethical considerations in the field.

REFERENCES

1. Bunzel R, Radford EJ, Hovatta O. Clinical and laboratory management of human ART: Keeping track of your data. J Assist Reprod Genet. 2014;31(9):1183-90.
2. Zegers-Hochschild F, Adamson GD, Dyer S, Racowsky C, de Mouzon J, Sokol R. The International Committee for Monitoring Assisted Reproductive Technology (ICMART): World report on assisted reproductive technology, 2014. Fertil Steril. 2017; 107(6):1583-91.
3. Riezzo I, Neri M, Bello S, Pomara C, Turillazzi E. Ethical and legal issues in reproductive health: Informed consent. Clin Exp Obstet Gynecol. 2013;40(3):437-41.
4. Ethics Committee of the American Society for Reproductive Medicine. Informed consent and the use of gametes and embryos for research. Fertil Steril. 2018;109(4): 825–9.
5. Hodson N, Daniels KR, Haimes E. Ensuring the confidentiality of donor-conceived individuals. Reprod Biomed Online. 2018; 37(1):31-38.
6. Pennings G, de Wert G, Shenfield F, Cohen J, Devroey P, Tarlatzis B; ESHRE Task Force on Ethics and Law. ESHRE task force on ethics and law: Gamete and embryo donation. Hum Reprod. 2017;32(10):1959-64.
7. Sills ES. Donor gametes and assisted reproductive technology: Legal frameworks and ethical considerations. Reprod Biomed Online. 2016;33(1):3-11.
8. Government of India. The Assisted Reproductive Technology (Regulation) Act, 2021. [online] https://dhr.gov.in/document/acts-circulars/assisted-reproductive-technology-regulation-act-2021 Available from [Last accessed November, 2024].
9. Schurr P, Wiegering V, Friese K. Surrogacy: The current situation and future perspectives. Geburtshilfe und Frauenheilkunde. 2020; 80(2):188-96.
10. Government of India. The Surrogacy (Regulation) Act, 2021. [online] https://dhr.gov.in/document/acts-circulars/surrogacy-regulation-act-2021 Available from [Last accessed November, 2024].

19 CHAPTER

Future Trends in Assisted Reproductive Technology

INTRODUCTION

The future of assisted reproductive technology (ART) is being shaped by groundbreaking innovations and emerging technologies aimed at improving success rates, accessibility, and outcomes. Techniques like gene editing, in vitro gametogenesis (IVG), and non-invasive embryo assessment are revolutionizing the field by offering more precise interventions and expanding possibilities for diverse populations. Innovations such as artificial intelligence (AI), nanotechnology, and time-lapse imaging further enhance embryo selection and personalized treatment planning. As ART continues to evolve, these advancements promise to address existing challenges while raising important ethical, societal, and regulatory considerations, ensuring responsible integration into clinical practice.

INNOVATIONS IN ASSISTED REPRODUCTIVE TECHNOLOGY

Emerging Technologies and Techniques

Assisted reproductive technology (ART) continues to evolve, driven by advances in medical science and technology. These innovations promise to enhance the efficacy and accessibility of ART, potentially revolutionizing the field **(Table 1)**.

Gene Editing and CRISPR-Cas9

Gene editing, particularly using CRISPR-Cas9 technology, holds transformative potential for ART. This technique allows precise modifications of the genome, which could be used to correct genetic disorders in embryos before implantation.[1] Although still in its infancy for clinical application, research suggests that CRISPR could significantly reduce the incidence of hereditary diseases. Studies have demonstrated its potential to correct mutations causing monogenic disorders, such as cystic fibrosis and sickle cell anemia.[2] However, challenges such as off-target effects and ethical concerns need to be addressed before widespread clinical use.[3]

Artificial Gametes

The development of artificial gametes through in vitro gametogenesis (IVG) is another promising frontier. This technology involves creating sperm and eggs from somatic cells, potentially aiding individuals with infertility issues who cannot produce viable gametes. Advances in IVG have shown that mouse stem cells can be reprogrammed to produce functional gametes, and efforts are underway to replicate these results in humans.[4] This breakthrough could also enable same-sex couples to have genetically related children and provide new options for cancer patients who become infertile due to treatments.[5]

TABLE 1: Upcoming technologies and their potential impact on assisted reproductive technology (ART).

Technology	*Description*	*Potential impact on ART*
Artificial intelligence (AI)	Use of AI algorithms to analyze data and improve decision-making in embryo selection and treatment plans	• Increased accuracy in embryo selection • Personalized treatment plans • Enhanced success rates • Reduced time and cost
CRISPR gene editing	Precise editing of genes to correct genetic disorders	• Potential to prevent hereditary diseases • Improved genetic health of embryos • Ethical and regulatory considerations
Organoids and 3D culture systems	Development of miniaturized, simplified versions of organs to study human development and disease	• Better understanding of embryo development • Improved culture conditions • Potential for personalized medicine
Time-lapse imaging	Continuous monitoring of embryo development without disturbing the culture environment	• Detailed observation of embryo development stages • Improved embryo selection • Increased implantation success rates
Microfluidics	Use of micro-scale devices to manipulate small volumes of fluids for sperm and embryo handling	• More precise handling and sorting of sperm and embryos • Reduced damage to gametes and embryos • Enhanced success rates
Bioprinting	3D printing of biological tissues and structures for reproductive medicine applications	• Potential for creating artificial ovaries and testes • Improved understanding of reproductive biology • New possibilities in fertility treatments
Nanotechnology	Application of nanoparticles for targeted delivery of drugs and imaging agents	• Targeted delivery of fertility drugs • Enhanced imaging for diagnostics • Potential for noninvasive treatments
Robotics	Use of robotic systems to assist in precise surgical and nonsurgical procedures	• Increased precision in procedures like intracytoplasmic sperm injection (ICSI) • Reduced human error • Enhanced outcomes in reproductive surgeries
Epigenetic modulators	Compounds that can modify the expression of genes without changing the DNA sequence	• Potential to improve embryo quality • Better understanding of gene expression in early development • Ethical and regulatory considerations

Noninvasive Embryo Assessment

Emerging noninvasive methods for embryo assessment, such as time-lapse imaging and metabolomic profiling, aim to improve embryo selection.[6] Time-lapse imaging allows continuous monitoring of embryo development, providing detailed insights into their growth patterns and viability without the need for invasive biopsies.[7] This technology has shown promise in improving implantation and pregnancy rates by identifying embryos with the best developmental potential.[8] Metabolomic profiling analyzes the biochemical environment of the embryo, offering another layer of assessment to enhance selection accuracy by identifying metabolic markers of embryo viability.[9]

Potential Impact on Assisted Reproductive Technology Outcomes

The integration of these emerging technologies into clinical practice could significantly impact ART outcomes:

- *Increased success rates:* Enhanced precision in genetic editing and embryo selection could lead to higher implantation and pregnancy rates, reducing the need for multiple IVF cycles.[8]
- *Reduced genetic disorders:* The ability to correct genetic abnormalities in embryos could decrease the prevalence of inherited diseases, leading to healthier offspring.[4]
- *Expanded access:* Technologies such as IVG could make ART accessible to a broader range of individuals, including those who are currently unable to produce viable gametes.[5]

ETHICAL AND SOCIETAL IMPLICATIONS

Ethical Considerations in Assisted Reproductive Technology

The rapid advancement of ART technologies brings significant ethical considerations that must be addressed.

Genetic Editing and Designer Babies

The potential use of gene editing in embryos raises concerns about the ethical implications of "designer babies", where genetic modifications could be used for nontherapeutic enhancements, such as selecting for desired physical or intellectual traits. This possibility necessitates strict ethical guidelines and regulations to prevent misuse and ensure that genetic interventions are limited to therapeutic purposes.[10] The debate includes concerns about equity, consent, and the long-term societal impacts of genetic modifications.[11]

Artificial Gametes and Reproductive Rights

The development of artificial gametes poses ethical questions about reproductive rights and the definition of parenthood. As IVG technology advances, ethical frameworks will need to address issues related to the rights of individuals to create gametes, the implications for donor anonymity, and the potential for creating embryos without a genetic mother or father.[12] There are also concerns about the commodification of human gametes and the potential psychological impacts on children born from such technologies.[13]

FUTURE DIRECTIONS AND CHALLENGES

The future of ART is likely to be shaped by ongoing technological innovations and the ethical frameworks that guide their implementation. The key directions and challenges include:

Regulatory Frameworks

Developing comprehensive regulatory frameworks will be essential to ensure the ethical use of new ART technologies. These frameworks should balance the potential benefits of innovations with the need to protect individuals and society from potential harms.[12] International cooperation and consensus will be crucial to address the global implications of these technologies.[14]

Accessibility and Equity

As ART technologies evolve, ensuring equitable access to these advances will be a significant challenge. Policymakers and healthcare providers must work to ensure that technological advancements do not exacerbate existing disparities in access to fertility treatments.[15] Efforts should be made to integrate new technologies into public healthcare systems and provide financial support for those who cannot afford expensive treatments.[16]

Societal Acceptance

The acceptance of new ART technologies by society will play a crucial role in their adoption and integration into clinical practice. Public engagement and education will be important to foster understanding and acceptance of these innovations, addressing misconceptions and ethical concerns.[17] Transparency in research and clinical applications, along with open dialogues about the benefits and risks, will help build public trust.[18]

CONCLUSION

The future of ART holds immense promise, driven by rapid technological advancements. However, the integration of these innovations into clinical practice must be carefully managed within ethical and regulatory frameworks to ensure they benefit individuals and society as a whole. Continued research, ethical vigilance, and public engagement will be essential to navigate the complexities and maximize the potential of these groundbreaking technologies.

REFERENCES

1. Liang P, Xu Y, Zhang X, Ding C, Huang R, Zhang Z, et al. CRISPR/Cas9-mediated gene editing in human tripronuclear zygotes. Protein Cell. 2015;6(5):363-72.
2. Doudna JA, Charpentier E. The new frontier of genome engineering with CRISPR-Cas9. Science. 2014;346(6213):1258096.
3. Ma H, Marti-Gutierrez N, Park SW, Wu J, Lee Y, Suzuki K, et al. Correction of a pathogenic gene mutation in human embryos. Nature. 2017;548(7668):413-9.
4. Hayashi K, Ogushi S, Kurimoto K, Shimamoto S, Ohta H, Saitou M. Offspring from oocytes derived from in vitro primordial germ cell-like cells in mice. Science. 2012;338(6109): 971-5.
5. Saitou M, Miyauchi H. Gametogenesis from pluripotent stem cells. Cell Stem Cell. 2016; 18(6):721-35.
6. Bromer JG, Yang Y, Lee A, Khan S, Park J, Seli E. Metabolomic profiling of human embryos: potential to improve outcomes. Reprod Biomed Online. 2012;24(2):146-53.
7. Wong CC, Loewke KE, Bossert NL, Behr B, De Jonge CJ, Baer TM, et al. Non-invasive imaging of human embryos before embryonic genome activation predicts development to the blastocyst stage. Nat Biotechnol. 2010;28(10):1115-21.
8. Rubio I, Kuhlmann R, Agerholm I, Kirk J, Herrero J, Escribá MJ, Bellver J, Meseguer M. Prospective evaluation of time-lapse imaging for preimplantation genetic screening: a pilot study. Fertil Steril. 2014;102(4):750-6.
9. Seli E. Metabolomics in embryo selection. Reprod Biomed Online. 2016; 32(1):22-30.
10. Savulescu J, Kahane G. The moral obligation to create children with the best chance of the best life. Bioethics. 2009;23(5):274-90.
11. Lanphier E, Urnov F, Haecker SE, Werner M, Smolenski J. Don't edit the human germ line. Nature. 2015;519(7544):410-1.
12. Baylis F. The ethics of creating children with three genetic parents. Reprod Biomed Online. 2013;26(6):531-4.
13. Palacios-González C, Harris J, Testa G. In vitro derived gametes and cloning: a challenge to

parental relationships and kinship. Reprod Biomed Online. 2014;29(6):647-54.

14. Isasi R, Kleiderman E, Knoppers BM. Editing policy to fit the genome? Science. 2016;351(6271):337-9.
15. Inhorn MC, Patrizio P. Infertility around the globe: new thinking on gender, reproductive technologies and global movements in the 21st century. Hum Reprod Update. 2015; 21(4):411-26.
16. Van Voorhis BJ. Clinical practice. In vitro fertilization. N Engl J Med. 2007;356(4):379-86.
17. Harper JC, Kennett D, Reisel D, Coonen E, Handyside AH. Global issues in assisted reproductive technology. Reprod Biomed Online. 2014;29(6):616-21.
18. Hendriks S, Boers SN, van der Bolt N, Bredenoord AL. Responsible research and innovation in genome editing. Reprod Biomed Online. 2016;33(4):410-21.

Index

Page numbers followed by *f* refer to figure and *t* refer to table.

E

F

G

H

I

K

L

M